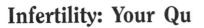

Infertility: Your Qu

Presented
with the
compliments
of

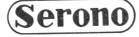

Serono Laboratories (UK) Limited
Welwyn Garden City, Herts AL7 1BG

NOTICE

Medicine is an ever-changing science. As new research and clinical experience broaden our knowledge, changes in treatment and drug therapy are required. The editors and the publisher of this work have checked with sources believed to be reliable in their efforts to provide information that is complete and generally in accord with the standards accepted at the time of publication. However, in view of the possibility of human error or changes in medical sciences, neither the editors, nor the publisher, nor any other party who has been involved in the preparation or publication of this work warrants that the information contained herein is in every respect accurate or complete. Readers should consult with their own physicians regarding particular conditions and treatments.

Infertility: Your Questions Answered

Seang Lin Tan
MBBS, MRCOG, MMed (O&G), AM
Senior Lecturer in Obstetrics and Gynaecology
Department of Obstetrics and Gynaecology
King's College School of Medicine and Dentistry
London SE58X
United Kingdom

Howard S Jacobs
MD, FRCP
Professor of Reproductive Endocrinology
University College and Middlesex School of Medicine
The Middlesex Hospital
London WIN 8AA
United Kingdom

McGRAW-HILL BOOK CO

Singapore   New York   St. Louis   San Francisco   Auckland
Bogotá   Caracas   Colorado Springs   Lisbon   London
Madrid   Mexico   Milan   Montreal   New Delhi   Oklahoma City
Panama   Paris   San Juan   Sydney   Tokyo   Toronto

Infertility: Your Questions Answered

1 2 3 4 5 6 7 8 9 0 KHL LG 9 5 4 3 2 1 0

ISBN 0-07-100619-2

This book was set in 10/12 Clearface Regular
Typeset by Linographic Services Pte Ltd

Printed in Singapore

Dedicated to our
wives
and to our
families

CONTENTS

ACKNOWLEDGEMENTS

It is a pleasure to acknowledge the help of our patients and colleagues for their many useful suggestions. Dr Machelle Seibel has been particularly helpful in this regard. While we feel that the book has benefited from these discussions, any errors are our own.

We particularly thank Ms Anita Patel for Figures 1.7A-C, 5.2A-C and 5.3A-B; Ms Judy Adams for Figures 5.4A-B and 5.5; Dr Christopher Steer for Figure 5.6A-B; Dr Angela Taylor for Figure 5.7A-B; Dr Machelle Siebel for Figures 5.9A-H and 5.10 and Dr Carla Mills for Figures 11.4 and 11.5.

We thank Mr Christopher Kenyon for drawing Figures 2.1, 2.2, 3.1A-C, 10.1, 11.6 and 13.2; Dr Gerard Conway for Figure 7.1 and Ms Sue Lee for all of the other diagrams.

ABOUT THE AUTHORS

Seang Lin Tan

Dr S L Tan is a graduate of the University of Singapore. He received his specialist training in Obstetrics and Gynaecology at the Kandang Kerbau Hospital in Singapore and his subspecialist training in Reproductive Endocrinology and Infertility in the Department of Reproductive Endocrinology at the Middlesex Hospital and the Department of Obstetrics and Gynaecology at King's College Hospital in London, where he is currently Senior Lecturer in Obstetrics and Gynaecology.

Dr Tan has had a brilliant academic career and has received numerous prizes and awards. He was awarded the MRCOG prize medal by the Royal College of Obstetricians and Gynaecologists in London as well as the Howard Eddey Gold Medal by the Royal Australasian College of Surgeons. He was also honoured with the Benjamin Henry Sheares Memorial Lectureship and Gold Medal by the Obstetrical and Gynaecological Society of Singapore and received the Obstetrics and Gynaecology Award from the Academy of Medicine for his research in Obstetrics and Gynaecology. He has published extensively on various aspects of infertility treatment and has more than 140 scientific publications and conference papers to his credit. He has lectured widely on different aspects of reproductive medicine and has been invited to speak at many international medical conferences. His previous books include "Pregnancy and Childbirth", "Frontiers in Reproductive Endocrinology and Infertility", "Advances in Reproductive and Perinatal Medicine" and "Recent Advances in the Management of Infertility". Dr Tan is married and has two children.

Howard S Jacobs

Professor Howard Jacobs is a world renowned authority in Reproductive Endocrinology and Infertility. After graduating from the University of Cambridge he trained in Endocrinology at the Middlesex Hospital Medical School in London and in Reproductive Endocrinology at the University of California in Los Angeles, United States of America. He has been a consultant reproductive endocrinologist since 1974 and was the first Professor of Reproductive Endocrinology to be appointed in the United Kingdom. At present he is Professor of Reproductive Endocrinology at the University College and the Middlesex School of Medicine and Consultant Endocrinologist to the Middlesex Hospital in London. He is chief examiner in medicine for the University College and the Middlesex School of Medicine.

Among his numerous scientific achievements, he pioneered the use of pulsatile LHRH treatment and published the first paper in the world describing the use of LHRH analogues for desensitising the pituitary gland prior to ovarian stimulation in IVF. Patients from all over the world have come to consult him for their infertility problems and over the past twenty years he has helped literally thousands of childless couples conceive. He has published more than 200 papers on various aspects of reproductive endocrinology and infertility and has edited three books on the subject. He has received numerous honours in his illustrious career including the prestigious Watson Smith Lectureship of the Royal College of Physicians and the Lettsomian Lectureship of the Medical Society of London. Two of his conference papers have been awarded prizes — one at the American Fertility Society and the other at the European Society for Human Reproduction and Embryology. He is regularly invited to speak at major international medical conferences and has lectured in every continent in the world. Among his many lecture tours he was recently visiting Professor at the University of Sydney in Australia and the University of Belgrade in Yugoslavia. He had the distinction of being conferred Honorary Membership by the Society of Obstetrics and Gynaecology of Israel.

Professor Jacobs has served on the editiorial boards of numerous international medical journals, he is a member of a multitude of committees including those of the International Society of Gynaecological Endocrinology of which he is a founder member, the British Fertility Society and the Section of Endocrinology of the Royal Society of Medicine. He was appointed a member of the Committee on Safety of Medicines of the United Kingdom and he is a previous member of the Medical Research Council Grants Committee. He is a Trustee of the British Infertility Counselling Association. He has regularly featured on radio and television programmes on infertility. Professor Jacobs is married with three children.

FOREWORD

During the past twenty years or so, there has been widespread discussion about infertility and its treatment. The number of couples afflicted with this suffering is increasing and the methods of treatment are constantly debated by doctors, scientists, politicians and others worried about the technical details of the methods and their ethical implications. Yet many ordinary men and women facing the problem merely wish to have a chance of achieving one of life's greatest gifts, a child of their own to establish a family in the simplest and most effective way. This dearest wish, this fundamental stake in their future, has been denied to them perhaps for years, and their despair rises with every passing month. They seek knowledge about their clinical problems, clear advice and counselling, and search for specialists who can provide their much needed medical care.

This book sets out to help them and others to understand what causes infertility, why it can become so intractable, how modern treatments have brought hope to so many couples, and some of the things that can go wrong during treatment. It aims to educate, to clarify complicated issues, and it succeeds admirably. Its authors give a clear and sympathetic account of the human reproductive system in men and women, of the malfunctions that prevent the production of eggs and spermatozoa or impair conception, and of the approaches to medical care now available to doctors to alleviate the problems of infertility. It is written in a simple and direct manner, in language easily understood by patients and the non-specialists, and the sections of each chapter are presented in clear sub-sections enabling a problem and its cure to be identified quickly and easily. Yet despite this simplicity, all the fundamental clinical problems are presented and discussed clearly, treatments are specified and described without avoiding the more difficult parts, and the potential complications are given in language clear enough for ordinary men and women to understand without any loss of medical authority by the authors.

This book should prove to be of immense value to the thousands of infertile couples in every country of the world. It should also be read by many others trying to understand why their children or friends are having difficulty conceiving a child, by professionals engaged in the care of their patients and by teachers or ethicists who need a broad and easily understood summary of this area of medicine. Teaching the wider public the issues and therapies involved in new forms of medicine is one of the most important means of bringing effective treatments to men and women in need of them, and the only way of enabling everyone involved in medical care to understand the difficulties faced by doctors trying to apply new methods of patient care.

Infertility: Your Questions Answered is a timely, welcome book aimed at a large audience and is certain to be a most valuable and novel contribution to the literature available in this field. The authors have done a service to their profession and to their patients. I give it my highest commendation and send my sympathy and best wishes to the many couples it is designed to help.

R G Edwards, CBE, PhD, DSc, FRCOG, FRS
Emeritus Professor
Cambridge University
Cambridge

INTRODUCTION

The realisation that something has gone wrong, that a pregnancy has not come along despite not using any form of contraception for several months, often brings with it a feeling of crisis - *Is there a problem? Can we do anything about it? Who should we talk to?* This book will try to answer the questions that keep flooding in, sometimes as part of that initial panic, sometimes during the course of the medical investigations and treatment that may become necessary.

The first question is what to do if you suspect a problem. We have no doubt that the first person to turn to is the family doctor. You may just need the reassurance of learning that it normally takes several months to get pregnant. On the other hand, after talking to you and your partner, your doctor may consider it appropriate to begin the process of examination and testing to try to find out why a pregnancy has not started yet. In Chapter 5 we describe when we think is the right time to go to the doctor and what you can expect at the first consultation.

At one level, the medical problem of infertility is simple. Although there are a number of different causes of infertility (Chapter 4), basically the doctor needs to know if the woman is releasing eggs at the normal rate (Chapter 1), if the man is producing sperm in the right amounts (Chapter 2) and whether the two are able to meet so the egg can be fertilised (Chapter 3). In practice, as described in Chapter 5, there are standard tests to establish whether these various processes are occurring normally. If it turns out that eggs are not being released (Chapter 7), that the sperm are not normal (Chapter 14) or that there is something stopping the two meeting (Chapters 10 and 13), the way forward declares itself. Each of these possibilities will suggest a particular line of treatment, each of which we describe in the later sections of the book. We also give as realistic an account as we can of the success rates of these treatments.

At a deeper level, the problems posed by a couple's infertility are subtle and poignant and need care, sympathy and time. At the very first consultation most couples are emotionally charged and very anxious. The fear that we may not be able to have a child can affect us in many ways: it may make us angry at the unfairness of it all — fertility is after all a natural right — jealous at the sight of new babies with their parents — the world now seems entirely populated by them — and sad because of our feeling of loss. For many couples, a speedy resolution of the fertility problem quickly resolves their emotional distress.

We recognise that for others, however, the process of investigation, referral to a specialist unit and treatment can become drawn out and begin to dominate their lives. Other issues come to the fore: sexual intercourse may change from something done to make love to a technique for making babies. Some of the tests seem to involve such personal aspects of life and to demand such precise scheduling that it may seem that sex for pleasure has given way entirely to sex as a job for procreation; moreover, for some couples it seems that a third party is constantly assessing performance and passing judgement on it. It is easy to see how all this can begin to erode self-confidence and make the couple feel they are losing control of their lives.

How do other couples cope with these consequences of infertility? For some it is enough to feel that something is at last being done and that experts are engaged in an understandable medical process to overcome an understandable medical problem. But the problem is that infertility presents some very unmedical problems too. An obvious one is that it can be very difficult and embarrassing to talk about the problem, even to close friends and family. So at the very time one might hope for support from family and friends many couples find they are trying to deal with their problems in isolation. Crucial decisions about careers, about life plans, even adoption, are often put off or become the subject of rumination rather than discussion.

What to do? For some, reading the last few paragraphs will have been the first time they have appreciated how widespread and normal is the distress that infertility causes. We hope it will be clear that the next step must be to find some way of breaking through the silence that seems to enclose the experience of infertility. The family doctor is an obvious starting point, both to gain medical information and to talk to about personal and emotional issues.

The next thing to consider is whether to make contact with an infertility counsellor. The major aim of counselling is to encourage people to express and to accept the feelings that accompany the crisis of their infertility. It is not that we think counselling will cure your fertility problem, rather that we hope it will make it easier to cope with and will help couples to feel that they are regaining control over their lives. We wish there were always specially trained infertility counsellors available. At some clinics they are and we encourage you to ask for an appointment with one. Moreover, even if your clinic does not have a counsellor on its staff, the request for the contact will serve to remind the doctors of the need to press for such a person to join the team. In Chapter 16 we describe some of the ways people try to cope with these aspects of their problem and we also give contact information for a number of self-help groups.

Finally, this book. In our experience, the majority of couples are so nervous at their initial consultations that few of the questions that they want answered get asked and few of the answers that are provided are remembered very well. Doctors have a regrettable tendency to lapse into jargon. Clinics are often rushed. We have written this book to answer the sorts of questions we have been asked over the last 15 years and to answer them in a way that we hope is detailed but clear. We have tried our best not to fudge issues and if, in our opinion, a particular test is not worth doing or a treatment not worth having we have said so. We do, however, recognise that in some clinical situations, medical opinions differ; in such cases, while giving our own advice we have also drawn attention to the controversy.

We do not expect that the whole book will be read by every person, for example, the woman who has blocked tubes will not want to read all about treatment to induce ovulation. Most people will find the first six chapters helpful; thereafter how much to read will depend on what your problem turns out to be and on what treatment you need. It is our hope that this book will complement the information you receive from the infertility specialists you consult and that it will provide you with information you can absorb in your own time, rather than in the limited time available in the consultation room.

1

REPRODUCTION IN WOMEN

1. Which are the female reproductive organs?

The female sex organs that are important for reproduction are the external genitalia, that is, the vulva, and the internal genitalia, namely the vagina, uterus, fallopian tubes and ovaries.

The vulva

This consists of several structures that surround the entrance to the vagina (Figure 1.1).

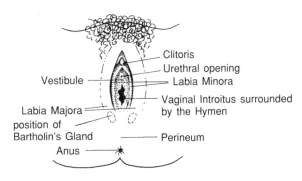

Figure 1.1 Female external genitalia.

The **labia majora** are two large folds of skin that surround the opening of the vagina. They contain fatty tissue, hair follicles and sweat glands. They form a pad of fat in front, called the mons pubis, which lies over the pubic bone. At the back, the labia majora merge with a number of muscles to form the perineal body, which lies between the vagina and anus.

The **labia minora** are the two delicate folds of skin which lie inside the labia majora on both sides of the entrance to the vagina. They contain a little connective tissue and many blood vessels.

1

The **clitoris**, developmentally equivalent to the penis, is normally about an inch (2.5 cm) long and consists of erectile tissue which becomes swollen with blood when a woman is sexually excited.

The **hymen** is a thin membrane that surrounds the opening of the vagina. Even in the virginal girl it is incomplete, so as to allow menstrual flow. The hymen is broken the first time sexual intercourse occurs but some remnants normally remain, even after repeated intercourse.

The **Bartholin's glands** are situated on either side of the vaginal passage. They secrete the mucus that provides lubrication during intercourse.

The Internal Genitalia
This consists of the vagina, uterus, fallopian tubes and ovaries (Figures 1.2 and 1.3).

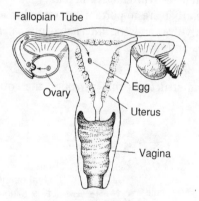

Figure 1.2 Female internal genitalia (front view).

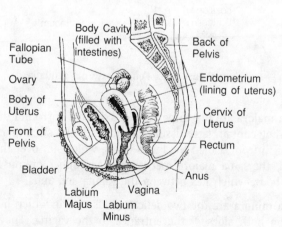

Figure 1.3 Side view of the female pelvis.

The **vagina** is the passage which leads from the vulva to the uterus. Its walls are lined by skin which contains many folds. The vagina is normally about 4 inches (10 cm) long but it stretches considerably during sexual intercourse and, of course, during childbirth.

The **uterus**, or womb, is a hollow pear-shaped organ measuring about 3 inches (7.5 cm) in length and 2 inches (5 cm) in width. It is divided into three parts — the fundus, the body and the cervix. The fundus is the top part, the body is the main middle portion and the cervix is the neck of the uterus. The uterus is lined by a specialised layer of tissue called the **endometrium** which thickens during the course of the ovulation cycle and is shed during menstruation (Chapter 1, question 8).

The **fallopian tubes** are two hollow tubes which project from the body of the uterus towards the ovaries. They are about 4.5 inches (11 cm) long and their outer ends hang over the ovaries with finger-like processes, called fimbriae. The tubes provide the connection between the ovaries and the inside of the uterus. They are lined with specialised cells which propel the egg towards the uterus once the egg has been picked up by the fimbriae.

Fertilisation of the egg and early development of the embryo take place in the fallopian tube. The egg passes from the tube into the uterus 60-70 hours after ovulation. This movement, which occurs in the reverse direction to that recently taken by the sperm, depends on the action of the delicate cells that line the fallopian tubes as well as muscular contractions of the tubes themselves.

The **ovaries** are almond-shaped, whitish structures normally located on the side walls of the pelvis. Each ovary is about 4 x 3 x 1 cm and consists of an outer layer called the cortex, which contains the eggs embedded in cells collectively called stroma, a central medulla and an inner hilar region through which blood vessels and nerves enter (Figure 1.4).

The ovaries are the female equivalent of the testes in men and besides contain-

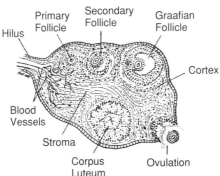

Figure 1.4   A schematic representation of a cross-section of the ovary.

ing the eggs they also produce a number of hormones, principally oestrogen and progesterone.

2. How many eggs is a woman born with?

The fetus has about seven million eggs during the fifth month of pregnancy. At birth, however, the ovaries contain only about 2 million eggs and by puberty about 400,000.

A woman is born with her full complement of eggs and no new ones are produced after birth.

3. What happens to them all?

The ovaries are in a resting state after birth but by the time of puberty, many of the eggs will have disappeared through a process called **atresia**, that is, the degeneration and eventual elimination of the egg cells. This process continues throughout life, even during pregnancy.

At the time of puberty, activation of the ovaries begins because the hypothalamus and pituitary gland start to release their hormones (see question 4). At the beginning of each ovulation cycle, about twenty eggs start to develop. As the cycle progresses, however, only one egg is selected to continue developing while the remainder degenerate.

Since one egg is usually ovulated each month only about 400 eggs are ovulated in a woman's lifetime. The rest of the eggs undergo atresia. The rate of atresia is determined by genetic as well as environmental factors, such as irradiation, certain drugs (Chapter 7, question 7) and cigarette smoking. When almost all the eggs have undergone atresia, menopause occurs.

4. What are the hormonal changes that take place in a normal menstrual cycle?

The sequence of hormonal changes that occur during each ovulation cycle is shown in Figures 1.5 and 1.6. There are two glands that produce the hormones that regulate ovulation. The upper gland, which is part of the brain, is called the **hypothalamus**. The hypothalamus secretes a hormone called **luteinising hormone releasing hormone (LHRH)** which stimulates the lower gland, the **pituitary**, to produce the hormones, **follicle stimulating hormone (FSH)** and **luteinising hormone (LH)**. Collectively FSH and LH are called **gonadotrophins**. LHRH is secreted in pulses and each pulse of LHRH leads to secretion of a pulse of the gonadotrophins. The time interval between each pulse varies with the phase of the cycle. During the follicular phase of the ovulation cycle (the first half, before ovulation occurs) LHRH is released every 1-1.5 hours. During the luteal phase (the second half, after ovulation occurs) the rate slows to one pulse every 4 hours.

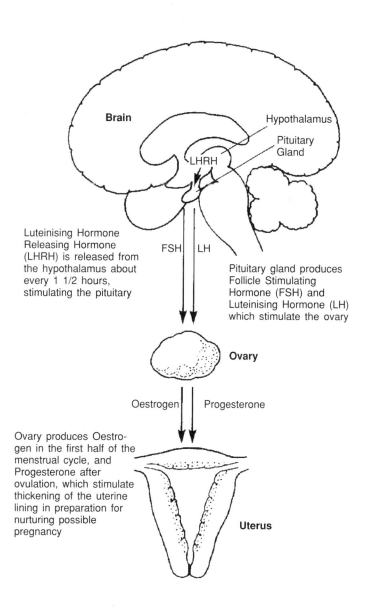

Figure 1.5 Hormonal control of the menstrual cycle.

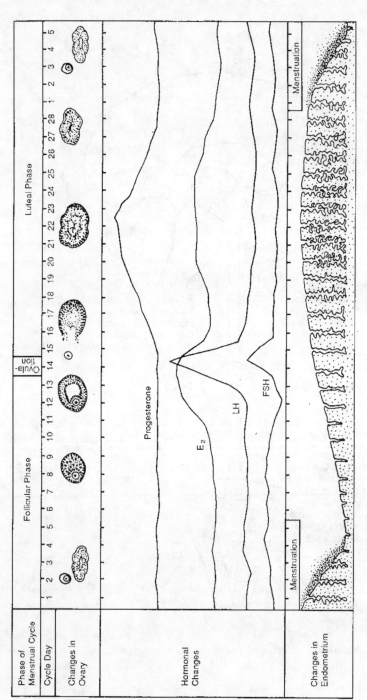

Figure 1.6 The normal menstrual cycle.

At the beginning of the cycle, that is, at the time of menstruation, blood levels of the hormone oestrogen are very low. In response to the low levels, the hypothalamus releases more LHRH that stimulates the pituitary gland to secrete more FSH. FSH stimulates the ovary and a number of follicles start to develop (the follicle is a fluid-filled sac which contains an egg and its surrounding cells). As the the follicles develop they secrete oestrogen and blood levels of oestrogen start to rise. One of the follicles, the one ultimately destined to ovulate, grows faster than the others and continues to produce increasing amounts of oestrogen. Oestrogen has a dampening effect on the hypothalamus and pituitary gland so that the level of FSH then starts to fall. When this happens, the other (non-dominant) follicles cannot grow but the largest, **the dominant follicle**, continues to grow because it has acquired the ability to respond to the falling levels of FSH. This process is a miniature "struggle for survival" just as occurs in other evolutionary processes. Success in this struggle means that only the "fittest" follicle survives to produce the egg that will get fertilised.

Oestrogen levels (in particular oestradiol) rise throughout the follicular phase and stimulate growth of the endometrium. As the concentration reaches a critical level, it leads to a sudden release of LH from the pituitary gland. This mid-cycle surge of LH causes maturation of the egg within the dominant follicle and then, 36 hours or so after the beginning of the surge, it triggers ovulation, that is, release of a mature egg that is ready to be fertilised. In a normal 28-day cycle (counting from the first day of menstruation until the day before the next menstrual flow begins), the mid-cycle LH surge occurs on about day 12 and ovulation on day 14.

Once ovulation has occurred, the empty follicle collapses to form a yellowish structure on the surface of the ovary, called a **corpus luteum**. The corpus luteum continues the secretion of oestrogen but also secretes another hormone, called **progesterone**. These two hormones act together to inhibit further release of FSH and LH by the pituitary gland. If a pregnancy occurs, the corpus luteum continues to produce progesterone and oestrogen and these hormones sustain the endometrium so menstruation does not occur.

After the third month of pregnancy, the corpus luteum wanes and for the remainder of pregnancy these hormones are made by the placenta. If a pregnancy does not occur, the corpus luteum begins to degenerate about 10 days after ovulation. The levels of the two hormones continue to fall so that approximately 2 weeks after ovulation the endometrium is shed (menstruation) and LHRH secretion increases again, so beginning a new cycle.

5.   How does the egg develop to a mature stage?

Each egg is contained in a fluid filled structure called a follicle. Growth of the ovarian follicle occurs in response to the hormonal changes described above. At the start of the menstrual cycle, the follicle is minute but at the time of ovulation, it has a diameter of 18-26 mm. This increase in size is due mainly to accumulation of fluid within the follicle. Growth of the ovarian follicle can be seen on serial ultrasound scans of the ovary (Figure 1.7A-C).

As the follicle starts to grow, the oocyte (egg) enlarges and in the 36 hours immediately before its release from the ovary, it undergoes a major process of maturation. This process is set in train by the mid-cycle surge of LH, which causes ovulation a few hours later. The mid-cycle surge of LH is, therefore, a most important hormonal link between the ovarian follicle, the pituitary gland and hypothalamus (the brain) and the egg.

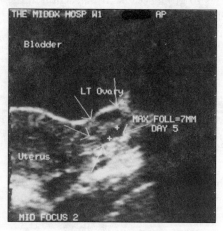

(a) Day 5 — follicullar diameter is 7 mm

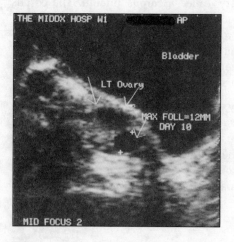

(b) Day 10 — follicular diameter is 12 mm

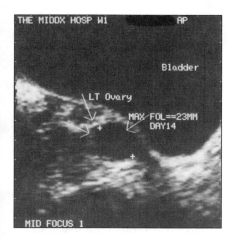

(c) Day 14 — follicular diameter is 23 mm

Figure 1.7 Growth of an ovarian follicle as seen on serial abdominal ultrasound scans.

6. How is the egg released?

The sudden rise in the level of LH at mid-cycle triggers ovulation. A tiny opening appears on the surface of the follicle, a little follicular fluid escapes and the egg is extruded and picked up by the fimbriae of the fallopian tube.

7. Does ovulation occur from alternate ovaries in alternate months?

No.

The chance of either ovary ovulating in any one month is entirely random. In any particular cycle it is not possible to know which ovary is going to ovulate until about 5 days before ovulation occurs. At this time an ultrasound scan will usually show which side the dominant follicle is on.

This question particularly concerns women who only have one healthy fallopian tube. Although it is believed that the tube is more likely to pick up eggs from the ovary next to it, we do know that it is possible for the tube to collect an egg that has come from the opposite ovary. This explains why some women who have only one ovary and a healthy tube on the opposite side can become pregnant.

8. What happens to the uterus during the menstrual cycle?

During the first half of the ovulation cycle, the **endometrium** (the lining of the uterus) is stimulated by the rising levels of oestrogen and becomes progressively thicker. This is called the **proliferative** phase. During the second half of the cycle, progesterone causes the endometrium to increase further in thickness. At the same time, the blood supply increases and the glands in the endometrium secrete a nutritious mucus, in preparation for implantation if the egg has been fertilised. This is called the **secretory** phase. If pregnancy does not occur, the corpus luteum degenerates, the levels of progesterone and oestrogen in the blood fall and the endometrium is shed. Menstruation has been likened to the "tears" of a frustrated uterus!

9. What do you mean by a regular menstrual cycle?
A regular menstrual cycle normally refers to a cycle which is 26-34 days long and whose length does not vary by more than 4 days from one cycle to the next.

10. If I have regular menstrual cycles does that mean I am ovulating?
Almost certainly.

Sometimes, however, an egg may develop partially without full maturation and release. In such cases, there will still be secretion of hormones and menstruation but the cycles are usually irregular.

11. What's the difference between the "ovulation" cycle and the "menstrual" cycle?
The "ovulation" cycle refers to the changes that take place in the ovary — the development of the dominant follicle, hence the term follicular phase, the process of ovulation at mid-cycle, followed by the development of a corpus luteum, hence the term luteal phase.

The "menstrual" cycle refers to the changes that take place in the uterus — the oestrogen induced growth of its endometrial lining, hence the term pro-liferative phase, followed after ovulation by the progesterone induced secretion of mucus from the endometrial glands, hence the term secretory phase.

2

REPRODUCTION IN MEN

1. Which are the male reproductive organs?
The male reproductive organs are the penis and testicles (Figure 2.1).

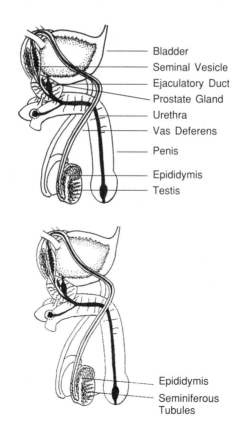

Bladder
Seminal Vesicle
Ejaculatory Duct
Prostate Gland
Urethra
Vas Deferens
Penis
Epididymis
Testis

Epididymis
Seminiferous
Tubules

Figure 2.1 Side view of male reproductive organs.

The **testicles** produce sperm and the male hormone, testosterone. Sperm are made in tiny tubes called **seminiferous tubules** which are coiled and packed tightly together. The tubules connect up to form bigger ducts which eventually join together into a single tube called the **epididymis**. The epididymis is tightly coiled too and if unravelled would be about 6 metres long. All the sperm travel through it. During their passage through the epididymis, sperm acquire the ability to move forward by themselves ("motility") and by the time they leave the epididymis, they are fully mature, motile and able to fertilise an egg. The epididymis joins to the **vas deferens**, a thicker tube that can be felt in the scrotum in most men.

The **penis** consists of spongy and erectile tissue and contains a channel called the **urethra** through which urine and sperm pass. The vas deferens fuses with the **seminal vesicle** (which makes some of the seminal fluid) to form the **ejaculatory duct** which passes through the **prostate gland** and opens into the urethra.

2. What are the hormones that affect reproduction in men?

The two pituitary hormones that affect reproduction in men are follicle stimulating hormone (FSH) and luteinising hormone (LH). They are exactly the same as the hormones of the same name that are found in women and, just as in women, they are secreted under the influence of LHRH produced by the hypothalamus.

In men, FSH stimulates the seminiferous tubules to produce sperm. LH stimulates specialised cells in the testes called **Leydig cells** to secrete the male hormone, testosterone. Besides producing the male characteristics, testosterone enhances the production of sperm.

The rate of LH secretion is influenced by the amount of testosterone circulating in the blood — if the testosterone levels fall then LH secretion increases in an attempt to return them to normal. FSH secretion is controlled by a recently characterised hormone called **inhibin**. The rate of inhibin secretion is governed by the amount of sperm being made by the seminiferous tubules. If sperm production falls, inhibin secretion falls too and so FSH levels rise.

3. How are sperm produced?

FSH and testosterone stimulate the germ cells (immature sperm) within the seminiferous tubules to divide and mature. The germ cells undergo various stages of development from spermatogonia to spermatid to spermatozoa (mature sperm). The appearance of a mature spermatozoon (sperm for short) is shown in Figure 2.2.

Each sperm has of a head which contains the chromosomes (containing the genetic material, the genes), a middle piece which supplies the energy for the

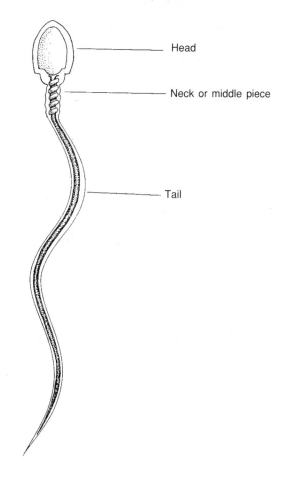

Figure 2.2 Mature spermatozoon.

sperm to swim and a tail which propels it through the female genital tract. Each sperm is about 0.05 mm long and so it can only be seen under the microscope.

One important difference between male and female reproduction is that, unlike the female who is born with her full complement of eggs, the male continuously produces sperm from the time of puberty.

4. How fast are the sperm produced?

It takes about 60 days for sperm to be produced and another 10-14 days for them to pass through the epididymis and vas deferens.

5.   What does semen contain besides sperm?
Essentially fluid from the seminal vesicles, the prostate and other glands which provides a vehicle to carry the sperm and at the same time helps to nourish them. The fluid is called seminal fluid.

6.   What happens at the time of ejaculation?
Ejaculation occurs as part of orgasm in men. The muscles at the base of the penis pump the seminal fluid forward in spurts. The volume of semen varies from 1-6 mls.

At the time of ejaculation the semen is thick but it liquefies inside the vagina within 20-30 minutes, through the action of enzymes produced by the prostate gland. The more active sperm penetrate the cervical mucus within 2 minutes of ejaculation and sperm have been found in the fallopian tubes 5 minutes after (artificial) insemination.

7.   How many sperm are released during intercourse?
On average 100-300 million sperm are deposited in the vagina at the time of ejaculation.

8.   Why are so many sperm released if only one is needed to fertilise the egg?
Because most die along the way.

A large number of sperm normally spill out of the vagina. Most remain in the cervical mucus and only about one in a thousand penetrates it. Some sperm are digested by cells that line the inside of the uterus and less than 200 reach the egg. While several may penetrate its outer covering, only one sperm succeeds in fusing with the egg. The sperm's struggle for survival parallels that of the egg and shows the fantastic care nature takes to try to ensure that only the fittest survive.

9.   How long do sperm survive inside the woman?
It is difficult to be sure.

Normally they survive for 2-4 hours in the vagina although motile sperm have been found there up to 16 hours after intercourse. Once the sperm enter the cervix, uterus or tubes, survival times are very variable. The average is 3-4 days although, rarely, sperm retain their fertilising ability for up to 7 days.

10.   Can I improve my sperm count by abstaining from sex?
No.

If the sperm are not ejaculated, they do not remain alive forever. After a while, they lose their fertilising ability and finally degenerate. If the sperm are not ejaculated for a long time, the proportion of older sperm in the semen increases so that, although the total sperm count may rise slightly, the semen quality does not improve. This is why abstaining from sex does not improve fertility.

11. Does illness affect the sperm count?
Yes.

Even an illness as simple as a sore throat for which you need treatment with antibiotics can depress the sperm count to zero. Since it takes about 70-74 days for production of new motile sperm, any illness during this time may affect sperm production. This is why it is important not to base a diagnosis on a single poor semen sample. Male infertility should only be diagnosed if repeated semen analyses over a few months reveal abnormal sperm counts or quality.

12. Do cigarette smoking and alcohol affect male fertility?
Yes.

Heavy cigarette smoking and consumption of alcohol adversely affect male fertility. Both the sperm count and motility are reduced by cigarette smoking. Although excessive alcohol consumption may reduce sperm production, its main effect is to impair testosterone secretion and accelerate its chemical breakdown and conversion to oestrogen. It, therefore, leads to reduced libido (sex drive). Alcoholism is also an important cause of impotence.

13. Does taking medications affect the sperm count?
A few medications such as salazopyrin (used to treat colitis), phenytoin (used to treat epilepsy), colchicine (used to treat gout), cimetidine (used to treat peptic ulcer) and nitrofurantoin (used to treat urinary infections) may reduce the sperm count. In each case there are alternative drugs that can be used that do not affect the sperm count and in each case the count recovers after the drug has been stopped.

Drugs used in the management of certain cancers, such as cyclophosphamide, may cause permanent infertility if used in large doses. They do not, however, seem to impair testosterone secretion.

14. Do narcotic drugs affect fertility?
Yes.

Marijuana has been found to cause infertility, probably by reducing the secretion of the hormones FSH and LH. Hard drugs, in particular morphine and heroin, are well known causes of both infertility and impotence. They stimulate the release of another hormone called prolactin which leads to impaired sperm production, reduced testosterone secretion and impotence.

15. What else affects sperm production and function?

The recognised causes of infertility in men are problems of sperm production, defective sperm transport, disorders of the accessory glands, and mechanical problems of intercourse or ejaculation.

Abnormal sperm production may be caused by a hormonal problem, undescended testicles or testicles that have been damaged by mumps (both testicles must have been affected to produce infertility), other infections or injury. **Varicocele** (Chapter 14, question 5), certain chemicals (for example, cadmium) and drugs sometimes damage the testes. In contrast to the situation in women, hormonal causes of infertility are unusual in men.

Obstruction of the ducts which transport sperm most commonly occurs as a result of infection or because of a congenital malformation in which the vas deferens is absent.

Inability to deposit semen into the female genital tract can result from impotence. If the opening of the penis is not at its tip, or if there is defective muscle control so that ejaculation of semen occurs into the bladder (**retrograde ejaculation**) instead of through its tip, problems arise that can usually be treated by a specialist urologist.

Unfortunately, in many cases of male infertility, no cause can be identified.

16. What are the figures for a normal sperm count?

A normal semen sample has a volume of between 1.5 and 6 mls, a sperm density of at least 20 million per ml, a progressive motility of at least 50 percent one hour after ejaculation and more than 60 percent of the sperm should have a normal shape (morphology). Sperm samples can, however, vary enormously and a diagnosis of male infertility should only be made if sperm tests are repeatedly abnormal.

17. What is the exact relation between fertility and the sperm count?

Obviously if the sperm count is zero (**azoospermia**) pregnancy cannot occur, unless the condition is temporary (see questions 11 and 13). It seems that the most important feature is the number of motile sperm that are in the ejaculate.

The generally accepted lower limit of normal for the total sperm count is 20 million per ml and fertility is reduced when the sperm count falls below this. It must be emphasised, however, that these figures are only a rough guide as it has been found that approximately 20 percent of men who have fathered a child have sperm counts lower than 20 million per ml.

3

GETTING PREGNANT

1.   How many sperm need to be ejaculated for pregnancy to occur?
No one knows exactly. In theory, only one is needed but most sperm die within the female genital tract before they reach the egg.

On average, men produce 200-300 million sperm each time they ejaculate. If the concentration is consistently below 20 million per ml the chances of pregnancy are reduced. Another point is that the motility (movement), morphology (structure) and fertilising capacity of the sperm are just as important as the number ejaculated.

2.   How and where do the sperm meet the egg?
Semen is initially thick and sticky but within 20-30 minutes of ejaculation it becomes liquefied by enzymes. Even before this occurs, some of the sperm that have landed closest to the cervix would have penetrated its mucus and we know that within 5 minutes of artificial insemination some very active sperm have reached the fallopian tubes!

Once the semen liquefies, many sperm quickly swim into the cervical mucus where they may remain for the next few days. A constant stream of sperm then swims up from the cervical mucus through the uterus into the fallopian tubes where they meet the egg in the outer half of the fallopian tube (the ampullary region, Figure 3.1A).

3.   How does fertilisation occur?
The human egg is covered by a jelly-like shell called **zona pellucida** which, in turn, is surrounded by a layer of cells called **corona radiata**. When the sperm meet the egg, many try to penetrate the zona pellucida. Normally, only one succeeds (Figure 3.1B). A chemical reaction then prevents other sperm from penetrating the zona.

The genetic material of the sperm (contained in 23 chromosomes) and of the

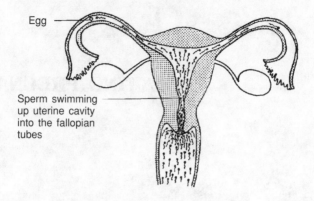

Egg

Sperm swimming
up uterine cavity
into the fallopian
tubes

Figure 3.1A Sperm swimming into the uterus and fallopian tubes.

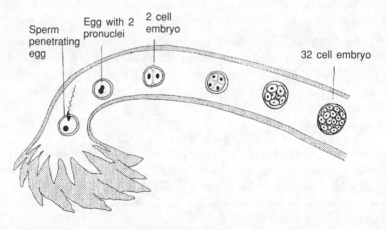

Sperm
penetrating
egg

Egg with 2
pronuclei

2 cell
embryo

32 cell embryo

Figure 3.1B A sperm fertilising the egg which then repeatedly divides.

egg (also contained in 23 chromosomes) then fuse. The fertilised egg, therefore, contains 46 chromosomes. If more than one sperm at a time could fertilise an egg, it would contain more chromosomes and, therefore, more genes from the father than the mother — a most unbalanced individual!

4. What happens to the egg after it is fertilised?
The fertilised egg is about 0.1 mm in diameter and over the next few days it repeatedly divides into two, four, eight, sixteen cells. Four days after fertilisation, it consists of a solid ball of cells called a **morula**, which is about 0.13 mm in diameter. The morula enlarges because of the accumulation of fluid inside it and develops into a **blastocyst**.

The blastocyst consists of a single layer of cells surrounding the fluid. A collection of cells forms a solid area on the inner side of the wall at one point. It is from this **inner cell mass** that the fetus subsequently develops.

Approximately 5 days after ovulation, the fertilised egg enters the uterus.

5. What is implantation? When does it occur?

Implantation refers to the burrowing of the blastocyst into the thickened secretory endometrium of the uterus (Figure 3.1C). It occurs about 7 days after fertilisation.

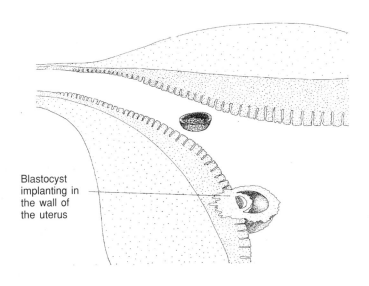

Blastocyst
implanting in
the wall of
the uterus

Figure 3.1C Blastocyst implanting in the wall of the uterus.

6. Can a woman get pregnant at any time of the menstrual cycle?

No.

One can only get pregnant around the time of ovulation, which is usually at mid-cycle. The time of ovulation may, however, be very variable.

7. How many days a month is a woman fertile?

Because sperm generally retain their fertilising capacity in the woman for about 48 hours after ejaculation and the egg can be fertilised for 24 hours after ovulation, the "fertile period" is normally about 3 days (that is, day 12-15 in a 28-day menstrual cycle). However, even in a woman with a 28-day menstrual cycle and with ovulation occurring on day 14, fertilisation can in rare cases occur from day 9 to day 15.

The "fertile period" therefore really refers to the phase of the cycle when the chances of pregnancy are best.

8. How can I find out when I am ovulating?
There are a number of ways.

You can keep a basal body temperature chart (Chapter 5, question 8), examine your cervical mucus (Chapter 5, question 24), have serial ultrasound scans to monitor the growth of the ovarian follicle (Chapter 5, question 13), use hormone urine test kits (Chapter 6, question 4) or have blood tests to detect the sudden rise of LH that occurs just before ovulation (Chapter 1, question 4).

9. Can we time sexual intercourse to improve our chances of pregnancy?
Yes, you can.

Since sperm survive longer after ejaculation inside the woman than does the egg after ovulation, you should aim to have intercourse just before ovulation occurs.

Here is a simple way to calculate the optimal time. The length of the second half of the menstrual cycle is more constant (around 14 days) than the first half, so keep a record of a few menstrual cycles. Supposing your shortest cycle in the past 6 months was 27 days and the longest 32 days, then ovulation is likely to occur in the present cycle anytime between day 13 (27 minus 14 days) and day 18 (32 minus 14 days), assuming that the length of the present cycle is more or less the same as the last few. Based on this calculation, it is a good idea to have intercourse about every other day from day 12 to day 19. This should ensure that no matter when ovulation occurs, there will be a pool of fertile sperm ready to fertilise the egg.

10. Does having sex too often reduce the chances of pregnancy?
No.

There is a myth that abstaining from sex until the fertile period enhances fertility. Although abstaining may slightly increase the sperm count, there is no evidence at all that abstinence is beneficial and it certainly goes against common sense. What is important is that sperm are in the vicinity of the egg when ovulation occurs.

For most couples, having intercourse every 36-48 hours around the time of ovulation gives the optimum chance of pregnancy.

11.   Is having an orgasm essential for conception?
No.

Fertility is not linked to the pleasure of sex. After all, pregnancy can occur as a result of artificial insemination.

12.   Is there a particular position during intercourse that is more likely to result in pregnancy?
No.

So long as semen is ejaculated into the vagina, there is no particular position that will increase the chances of pregnancy.

13.   ɪ think most of the semen flows out from my vagina after intercourse. Will this prevent me from getting pregnant?
No.

Semen liquefies after 20-30 minutes so some is bound to flow out. This does not matter because the active sperm penetrate the cervical mucus very quickly.

14.   Do I need to lie down for a certain period of time after intercourse to increase the chance of pregnancy?
No.

Movement of the sperm into the cervical mucus does not depend on the woman maintaining any particular position.

15.   Does pregnancy always occur if you have intercourse at the right time?
No.

The chance of pregnancy in any one cycle is about 15-25 percent even if the couple is perfectly fertile and is having intercourse at the right time. It is important to remember, therefore, that even when every factor is optimal, 75-85 percent of ovulatory cycles will not end in a pregnancy.

16.   What is a D & C? Does it help a woman get pregnant?
D & C stands for dilatation and curettage.

In this procedure, the passage through the cervix is dilated (widened) to allow a fine instrument called a curette to be passed into the uterus. This allows some of the endometrial lining to be removed, usually for examination under a microscope. It does not help the woman get pregnant except indirectly if it helps to establish the cause of infertility.

17.   What is an HSG? Does it help a woman get pregnant?
An HSG is a hysterosalpingogram, that is, an X-ray picture (gram) of the uterus (hystero) and fallopian tubes (salpingo).

Some doctors used to believe that it helped women who had mildly blocked fallopian tubes to conceive because the dye injected into the uterus at the time of the HSG "opened up" the fallopian tubes. There is, however, no good evidence to support this. An HSG only helps indirectly in the sense that it may help determine the cause of infertility so that appropriate treatment can be given.

18.   Does taking thyroid hormones help a woman get pregnant?
No, not unless blood tests and other investigations have proven that the thyroid gland is not functioning properly.

19.   What changes occur in a woman's body when she becomes pregnant?
Structural, functional and psychological changes occur and they are nature's way of preparing the woman for pregnancy and childbirth. The changes are temporary.

The breasts enlarge, the nipples become more prominent, the area surrounding the nipple (areola) becomes darkened and the veins over the breasts become more prominent. The uterus progressively increases in size. The circulating blood volume increases by 40 percent during pregnancy and the pulse rate rises because the heart has to work harder. As a result of the hormonal changes during pregnancy, some women may notice increased pigmentation on the face and a dark line appearing down the middle of the lower abdomen. The women's weight gradually increases, especially in the second half of pregnancy.

4

NORMAL FERTILITY AND THE CAUSES OF INFERTILITY

1.   How long does it take the average woman to get pregnant?
On average, a normally fertile couple, aged about 25, who are having regular sexual intercourse have a 25 percent chance of conceiving each month. Most such couples will, therefore, have achieved a pregnancy within a year of stopping contraception.

2.   What exactly do you mean by "infertility"?
Strictly speaking, an **infertile** patient is one who has no chance of getting pregnant without some medical assistance. In reality, few patients are completely infertile and most are **subfertile**, in the sense that they have a reduced chance of getting pregnant. For example, the chance might be 5 percent per cycle, rather than the 25 percent mentioned above.

However, because the word "infertility" is so widely used, it has come to mean the same thing as "subfertility" and that is the sense in which we use it in this book.

In general, patients are classified as "infertile" or "subfertile" if pregnancy has not occurred after 1 year of regular, unprotected sexual intercourse (that is, no contraception has been used).

3.   Do women become less fertile as they get older?
Yes, they do.

It has been estimated that a normal woman aged 25 years or younger takes on average 2-3 months to get pregnant compared with 6 months or more for a woman of 35 years or older. In the same way, if we study women who are having artificial insemination with donor semen, the monthly chance of a pregnancy is about 11 percent for women aged 25 years or younger but is reduced to 6.5 percent for women who are aged 35 years or older.

4. Why does this occur?

There are several reasons.

The first reason is that the eggs themselves age. Women are born with a fixed number of eggs and, unlike the situation in men, the germ cells in women never divide (germ cells refers to the eggs and the sperm). This means that an egg that is ovulated this month has been in the body, virtually unchanged, for the whole of the woman's life. A woman of 40 is therefore ovulating eggs that are themselves 40 years old. Such eggs may not be so easily fertilisable as eggs from younger women.

Second, women who are older are more likely to have abnormal embryos. The result is to impair implantation and increase the rate of miscarriage.

Third, as a result of atresia (Chapter 1, question 3), there is a progressive decline in the number of follicles and eggs in the ovary; there is also a steady increase with age of the proportion of menstrual cycles that are anovulatory.

Fourth, there is evidence that the endometrium is not so receptive as women age and so the chances of a normal embryo implanting are somewhat reduced on this account.

Fifth, there is a higher incidence of endometriosis (Chapter 9, question 1) and fibroids (Chapter 13, question 2) with increasing age and these may also impair fertility.

Finally, there may be a decline in the frequency of sexual intercourse with age.

It is important to appreciate that these are general points and many normal children are regularly born to women who are older than the average age at which women usually conceive.

5. Do men become less fertile as they get older?

Yes. However, the decline in male fertility with age is small and generally occurs after the age of 60 years.

6. What are the common causes of infertility?

Infertility may be caused by problems in men, in women or in both. In about 30 percent of cases the causes are purely male, in about 30 percent the causes are purely female and in the remainder there are problems on both sides.

The man may produce no sperm, too few, immotile or abnormal sperm. He might be impotent, or suffer from premature or retrograde ejaculation (Chapter 14, question 2).

The woman may not ovulate or ovulate infrequently. She may have blocked tubes, endometriosis, or abnormalities in the uterus such as fibroids.

As a couple, the cervical mucus may be hostile to the husband's sperm because of the presence of antibodies to the sperm (Chapter 13, question 7). Finally, there may be sexual problems that result in the sperm and the egg not meeting.

7.   Is infertility getting more common?
The answer is probably yes.

There are a number of reasons. Many women are getting married at an older age and once they are married they are more likely to delay having children. Sexually transmitted diseases are more common nowadays and many individuals have more sexual partners than in the past so they run a greater risk of transmitting or acquiring infections. These infections may produce pelvic inflammatory disease which, in turn, causes blocked fallopian tubes (Chapter 10, question 1).

Several recent surveys have indicated that about one in every six marriages has a fertility problem.

8.   Does a retroverted uterus or tilted womb cause infertility?
Eighty percent of normal women have an anteverted uterus (tilted forwards) while the rest have a retroverted uterus (tilted backwards). This is perfectly normal, just as most of us are right handed while it is quite normal to be left handed.

A retroverted uterus is only related to infertility if it is immobilised in that position by pelvic inflammatory disease or endometriosis.

9.   Does obesity cause infertility?
No, most obese women are fertile. However, obesity may be associated with polycystic ovary syndrome and abnormal hormone production (Chapter 7, question 34) which can cause infrequent ovulation. Being overweight does makes polycystic ovary syndrome worse.

10.   I have been told that women who take the birth control pill may have difficulty getting pregnant when they stop it. Is that true?
It may take women a few months longer to conceive after stopping the birth control pill compared with stopping contraception with the diaphragm. The effect is more noticeable in women in their late 30s than in younger woman. The effect is only temporary and has not been found in all studies. However, if a woman has been taking the pill primarily to treat a hormonal problem and not for birth control, the original hormonal problem may recur once treatment with the birth control pill is stopped.

It used to be thought that women who took the pill for many years had a higher risk of having no periods when they stopped the pill. This is not true at all. The reason why some women suddenly stop menstruating when they stop the pill is because they have developed some condition such as severe weight loss, premature menopause (Chapter 7, question 6) or raised prolactin levels (Chapter 7, question 19) while they were taking the pill. If they had not been on the pill they would have stopped menstruating earlier.

With regard to pelvic inflammatory disease (Chapter 10, question 1), it has been found that use of the combined contraceptive pill is associated with a 50 percent reduction in the incidence of this important cause of infertility. It is probably the progestogen component of the pill that reduces the penetrability of the cervical mucus to the types of bacteria that cause pelvic infection.

11. Do women who have used IUCDs for contraception find it more difficult to conceive?
Women who use IUCDs (intra-uterine contraceptive devices) have a slightly higher risk of developing pelvic inflammatory disease which may lead to blocked tubes. Otherwise there is no relation between IUCDs and infertility.

12. Does stress cause infertility?
There have been no valid experiments proving that stress itself causes infertility. It only does so if it is part of a condition like anorexia nervosa which causes the woman not to ovulate (Chapter 7, question 13). If the stress is sufficiently severe to reduce the frequency of sexual intercourse drastically then of course it does contribute to infertility.

Stress is certainly not a common or important cause of infertility.

Stress is, however, almost always an important and distressing consequence of infertility.

13. Does taking a holiday improve the chances of conception?
At some time or another, nearly all couples wonder whether it is stress that is causing their infertility. This is especially so when no obvious cause has been found. The case for stress as a cause of infertility is, however, weak.

Having said this, if the problems associated with infertility and its treatment are becoming overwhelming, it may be well worth taking a break from your routine. All infertility specialists have seen couples who conceived when they are on holiday or, indeed, when they have given up trying to have a child.

14. What are the chances of pregnancy for a couple attending an infertility clinic?
It is very difficult to give a precise figure because the success rate depends to a large extent on the type of patients that come to the clinic. Failure of

ovulation, for example, is much more successfully treated than tubal disease so a clinic which has mainly patients with ovulatory problems is more likely to have a good success rate than one which specialises in tubal problems.

Having said that, a large clinic which provides good infertility treatment and which sees the whole range of fertility problems will probably achieve a 50-60 percent pregnancy rate in patients followed up for 2 years.

15. What is meant by the term "cumulative conception rate"?

Cumulative conception rate is a statistical method of expressing the success rate of infertility treatment which takes into account treatment success and failure as well as patients who discontinue treatment for one reason or another. It also copes with different rates of follow-up.

The cumulative conception rate gives an estimate of what the pregnancy rate would have been if all patients were followed up for the same length of time. For example, a cumulative conception rate of 60 percent at 3 months means that 60 percent of all patients would be pregnant after 3 months of treatment. Calculation of cumulative conception rates allows us to compare the efficacy of different methods of treatment.

5

INVESTIGATION OF INFERTILITY IN MEN AND WOMEN

1. How long should we have tried for a child before seeking help?
Since the average fertile couple has about a 20 percent chance of conceiving each month, more than half of them will have achieved a pregnancy in 6 months and most within a year. As a guide, therefore, if you have been having intercourse regularly for 18 months without contraception and pregnancy has not occurred, you should seek medical advice.

2. When should a couple seek help earlier than this?
There are two categories of people who should seek help sooner.

First, couples who have some reason to suspect a problem - for example, if the woman is not having periods or if the cycle is very irregular (suggesting an ovulatory disorder), if there is a history of a pelvic infection or burst appendix (suggesting a possible tubal problem: Chapter 10, question 1) or if the woman experiences pain throughout the period or during intercourse (suggesting the possibility of endometriosis: Chapter 9, question 1).

Second, women over the age of 35. Two reasons: fertility declines with age (Chapter 4, question 3) so it is a good idea to seek help at an earlier stage to ensure the best chance of pregnancy. Second: fewer years are left if treatment is needed.

If you fall into the first category, we would advise you to consult your doctor straight away. If in the second category, we would advise you to try for a year before starting tests.

3. Do both of us have to go and see the doctor?
Infertility is a problem of a couple who are unable to have a child together. Since the problem could be in you, your partner or both of you, it is important that both of you should be examined at the same time.

4. What sort of questions will the doctor ask?

Doctors vary (thank goodness!) but, in general, they will ask you questions both as individuals and as a couple.

The woman

The doctor will probably start by asking your age, about how long you have been trying to have a baby in this and in any previous relationship, and about your menstrual periods - how old you were when they began, whether they are regular, how long they last and what kind of pain, if any, you have with them. You will also be asked about the length of your menstrual cycles and so, if you can, bring along a record of the dates of your periods for the last 6 months.

Next, there will be questions about whether you have any symptoms of ovulation, such as pain, watery cervical mucus and mild vaginal bleeding at mid-cycle. Any history that suggests the possibility of blocked tubes is important and this includes a history of sexually transmitted diseases, previous pelvic infection, appendicitis or any abdominal operation.

If you have any symptoms that may suggest endometriosis, such as pain deep inside the vagina during intercourse or pain during your periods that lasts the entire duration of menstrual flow, you should mention it now.

You should also tell your doctor if you have any other major illness or if you are on any medication.

The man

The doctor will probably ask about your general health, any previous major illnesses or operations. Operations or injury to the testicles or mumps (especially after puberty) may reduce sperm production. If you had pain in your testicles or sexually transmitted disease in the past you should tell your doctor as infections increase the risk that the sperm ducts are blocked.

You should also mention whether you are taking any regular medication (Chapter 14, question 2).

The couple

As a couple you will probably be asked how often you are having intercourse, whether you have tried to time it to coincide with any particular phase of the menstrual cycle and whether there are any sexual problems, such as premature ejaculation (ejaculation of semen before the penis is in the vagina).

We hope you will be asked about smoking: it impairs fertility in men and women, impairs the baby's development during pregnancy and is bad for the newborn baby's lungs. Now is the time to stop!

5. Do we have to be examined?

Yes. A physical examination is part of the evaluation and that includes a pelvic or internal examination for the woman and an examination of the man.

Pelvic examination
The doctor begins by examining the genital area, looking for any signs of hormonal disturbance or infection. An instrument called a speculum is then gently passed into the vagina. This enables the doctor to have a look at the cervix and vaginal walls. If you have not recently had a PAP smear, one will probably be taken now. This involves lightly scraping the cervix with a flattened piece of wood called a spatula (it resembles an ice-cream stick). The cells on the spatula are then wiped onto a glass slide which is sent to the laboratory to be examined under a microscope.

After the speculum is removed, the doctor inserts the gloved index and middle fingers into the vagina and places the other hand over the lower abdomen. By moving both hands the doctor can then feel the shape, size, position and mobility of the uterus and also whether there are any large cysts in the ovary or abnormal masses in the pelvis.

The man
The doctor will examine the testicles, paying particular attention to their size and consistency, to whether there are any lumps on them and whether there is a **varicocele**. A varicocele is a collection of swollen (varicose) veins, usually on the left side, which can only be diagnosed when the man is standing up. The penis is examined to see if there is any infection and whether the urethra opens normally at the tip.

6.   How do I know if I ovulate?
If you have regular menstrual cycles, especially if you get some premenstrual tension and mid-cycle pain, you are most likely to be ovulating. A good sign of ovulation is a watery cervical mucus. What you may notice is a little sticky discharge from the vagina which becomes increasingly watery as mid-cycle approaches. This is caused by the rising level of oestrogen that is produced by the enlarging ovarian follicle. Once ovulation has occurred the cervical mucus becomes thick again.

7.   What tests can be done to see if I am ovulating?
The usual tests performed are the basal body temperature chart (BBT), serial ultrasound scans of the ovaries, a biopsy of the endometrium and a blood test for progesterone.

8.   How do I keep a temperature chart?
The basal body temperature is the body's temperature when you wake up after a good night's sleep. A sensitive thermometer is needed, which you can buy from the chemist. Your temperature has to be measured every morning from

the beginning of your menstrual cycle. For women working on night shifts, the time to record the temperature is on waking up after a sleep of at least 4 hours.

You should keep the thermometer by your bed and check your temperature as soon as you wake up, before you get out of bed. Place the thermometer under your tongue for 3 minutes. Eating, drinking, washing your mouth or even moving about will change your body temperature.

You should record your temperature every day, until your period comes again, on a basal body temperature (BBT) chart (Figures 5.1A-E) which you can buy from the chemist or obtain from your doctor.

a)   Normal ovulatory pattern — there is a sharp rise in basal body temperature after ovulation.

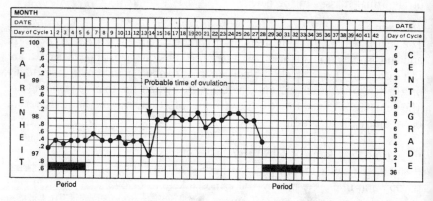

b)   Anovulatory pattern — the basal body temperature shows no significant change through the menstrual cycle.

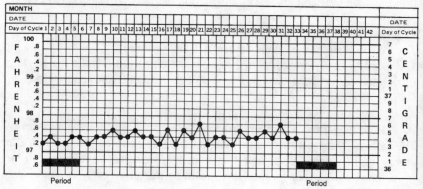

c) Stepwise rise in temperature is still indicative of ovulation but makes the day of ovulation difficult to anticipate.

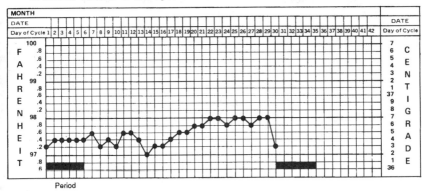

Period

(d) Short luteal phase — the internal between the temperature shift and menstruation is less than 10 days.

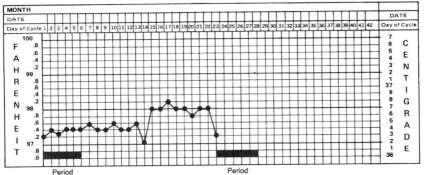

Period   Period

(e) Persistent elevation of the basal body temperature may be the first indication of pregnancy.

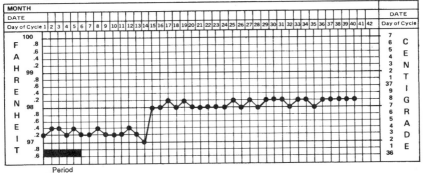

Period

Figure 5.1 Different patterns that may be seen on the basal body temperature (BBT) chart.

9. What does the basal body temperature chart show?

If you plot your basal body temperature for the entire menstrual cycle you will notice that, when the cycle is ovulatory, the temperature is higher in the second than in the first half of the cycle. The difference is usually about 1-1.5°C.

Figure 5.1A shows a BBT chart that suggests that ovulation has occurred. As you can see, the temperature does fluctuate a little from day to day. In an ovulatory cycle, the temperature may dip on the actual day of ovulation (although that often does not happen) but it rises sharply thereafter. The rise occurs through the action of progesterone, secreted by the corpus luteum. The rise in the temperature is maintained until a day or so before menstruation starts. This pattern of temperature on a BBT chart is called "biphasic".

In a cycle in which pregnancy occurs, the temperature remains elevated. In a cycle in which ovulation has not occurred (an anovulatory cycle) the temperature chart remains flat (monophasic: Figure 5.1B).

10. Is the basal body temperature chart reliable?

Frankly, not very.

There are a number of reasons. First, the temperature may not be recorded accurately. The woman may have a fever (although this should be recorded on the chart). Even if there is ovulation, the temperature pattern is rarely as perfect as described. The rise in temperature may be stepwise (Figure 5.1C) but provided that it is maintained for 12 days or more, the pattern is not important.

Another possibility is that the ovaries may not be working properly even though ovulation has occurred. If this happens, the temperature rise may not last the usual 12–14 days. When it is for less than 10 days it is called a "short luteal phase" (Figure 5.1D). Finally, some women are not very sensitive to progesterone so that even though they are ovulating, they do not have a rise of temperature on the BBT.

11. Can we use the BBT to tell us when ovulation occurs so we can time sexual intercourse accurately?

No.

A biphasic BBT chart only tells you that ovulation has occurred. Since it depends on progesterone from the corpus luteum elevating the temperature, it is no use for predicting ovulation, which occurs before the corpus luteum is formed.

12. So what are the practical uses of the BBT?

First, it is an inexpensive method which the woman can use herself to tell if ovulation is occurring. Second, it allows the doctor looking at the BBT chart to see (retrospectively) if you have had sex at the right time each month (you should record the days you have sex on the BBT chart). Finally, if the temperature rise continues for more than 14 days it may be the first sign of a pregnancy (Figure 5.1E).

But many couples become slaves to the temperature chart and the continual emphasis on timing can wreck the pleasure of sex. So, given their essential limitations (even when experts look at them they disagree on the interpretation of every fifth chart), we do not advise you to use them for too long. A couple of months provides as much useful information as does 6 months worth of records.

13. What is ultrasound scanning of the ovaries?

An ultrasound scan is a method of examining the internal organs of the body using high frequency sound waves. The images these sound waves provide look very similar to X-rays but they have the great advantage that, unlike X-rays, they do not damage the body's tissues.

For infertility work, two types of scans are used.

The first one that was used was the **abdominal** ultrasound scan. For this type of scan, the patient needs to have a full bladder. A small scan probe is placed over the lower part of the abdomen. The probe sends out small pulses of high frequency sound waves. These sound waves, which cannot be felt, bounce off the internal organs and are reflected back visually to be displayed on a television screen. The ultrasound machine is computerised, which allows the operator to "zoom in" on the ovaries and to take accurate measurements of the follicles. In the same way, the size of the uterus and the thickness of its endometrial lining can be measured.

The second type of scan is the **vaginal** ultrasound scan (see questions 16 and 17).

14. Is any special preparation needed for an ultrasound scan?

For an abdominal ultrasound scan, you need to have a full bladder, so you will be asked to drink 6–8 glasses of water an hour or so before the scan is due. It is also helpful if you can avoid high fibre food for about 3 days before the scan is performed.

It is generally said of a woman having an abdominal ultrasound scan, that if she is still smiling she has not drunk enough!

15. Why is a full bladder so important?

There are two reasons.

First, the abdominal wall and bowel (which contains air) conduct sound waves poorly so that the structures behind, namely the uterus and ovaries, cannot be seen. The full bladder not only pushes the surrounding bowel away but, more importantly, acts as a "window" through which sound waves can pass and the ovaries and uterus visualised.

Second, the best images are obtained when the organ being scanned is at right angles to the ultrasound beam. The uterus and ovaries are therefore optimally viewed when the bladder is distended.

16. I find having a very full bladder the worst part of the test. Is there any method of having an ultrasound scan without the need for a full bladder?

Yes, there is.

This is by doing a **vaginal** ultrasound scan. A small probe is placed in the vagina and it allows the uterus and ovaries to be scanned without a full bladder being necessary.

17. What are the advantages of doing a vaginal ultrasound scan compared with an abdominal one?

The main advantage of the vaginal scan is that the pictures of the ovaries and uterus are usually larger and clearer than those produced by the abdominal scan so the measurements taken are more accurate. This is because the ovaries and uterus are closer to the vaginally placed ultrasound probe and so the sound waves do not have to pass through so much tissue. The other advantage is that the scan can be done without any preparation, the patient does not need to have a full bladder and so there is less sense of urgency about the procedure.

Having said that, the abdominal scan produces pictures that are quite good enough in most cases, so if you are uncomfortable with the idea of a vaginal scan the abdominal approach is perfectly acceptable. Actually the vaginal scan does have its limitations — in a small number of cases the ovaries are located high in the pelvis, out of the focal zone of the probe and so they are inaccessible to transvaginal ultrasound.

In many infertility clinics both methods of scanning are available so the choice can be made by the patient.

18. How often must ultrasound scans be done to see if there is ovulation?

Usually a baseline scan is done on the second or third day of the cycle to allow the structure of the ovaries to be seen; solitary cysts in the ovary and polycystic ovaries can be diagnosed.

If the patient is not receiving any medication to stimulate multiple ovulation, the next scan is scheduled around day 10 of the cycle and by this time a dominant follicle should be visible. Once a follicle gets to about 12 mm in diameter it grows at a rate of about 2 mm a day. Ultrasound scans are then performed every other day until ovulation occurs.

19. What are the signs of ovulation on ultrasound?

In an ovulatory cycle, the dominant follicle grows until it has an average diameter of 18-26 mm (there is a range of follicle sizes when ovulation occurs). It then disappears and, on a subsequent scan, a solid corpus luteum can be seen in its place. There may also be a small amount of fluid seen at the back of the uterus (Pouch of Douglas) which comes from the ruptured follicle (Figure 1.7A-C — abdominal scans, Figure 5.2A-C — vaginal scans).

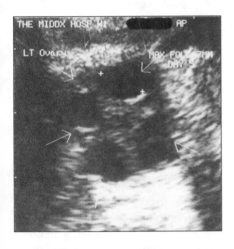

(a) Day 5 — follicular diameter is 7 mm

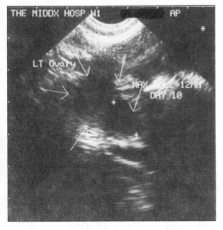

(b) Day 10 — follicular diameter is 12 mm

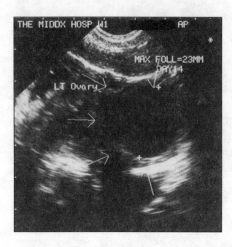

(c) Day 14 — follicular diameter is 23 mm

Figure 5.2 Growth of an ovarian follicle as seen on serial vaginal ultrasound scans.

The uterus enlarges and the endometrium thickens during the proliferative phase, in response to the secretion of oestrogen by the dominant follicle. After ovulation, the appearance of the endometrial echo changes in response to secretion of progesterone by the corpus luteum.

20. Does ovulation always occur once a dominant follicle has formed?
Usually.

But, it does not always happen, which is why serial ultrasound scans have to be performed. Sometimes there is inadequate stimulation, the follicle grows until it has an average diameter of 13-14 mm but then stops growing. In other cases there is no spontaneous mid-cycle LH surge so that although the follicle grows to a diameter of 20 mm or so it does not ovulate (Chapter 8, question 11). Finally, the follicle may not ovulate but continue to grow into a cyst instead (such cysts are not dangerous and disappear without any treatment being necessary).

21. What are the other uses of ultrasound in the investigation of infertility?
Ultrasound can be very helpful for diagnosing the cause of infertility. For example, it can suggest that there is an endometriotic cyst in the ovary or a hydrosalpinx, which is a collection of fluid in a blocked fallopian tube.

In patients with amenorrhoea who do not ovulate in response to treatment with clomiphene or tamoxifen (Chapter 8, question 12), ultrasound scanning can reveal three different types of picture.

The first is that seen in patients with **hypogonadotrophic hypogonadism** (Chapter 7, question 11). The ovaries are smaller than normal and show few follicles (Figure 5.3A). The uterus is small and the endometrium thin (Figure 5.3B). Such an image is also seen in patients with premature ovarian failure, although the two conditions are readily distinguished by hormone measurements.

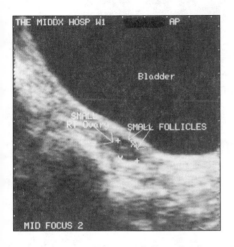

Figure 5.3A The ovary in a patient with hypogonadotrophic hypogonadism is small with no follicular activity.

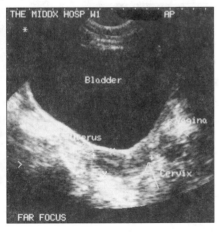

Figure 5.3B This shows a very small uterus in a patient with hypogonadotrophic hypogonadism.

The second picture is that seen in patients with **polycystic ovary syndrome**. These patients have ovaries that are usually larger than normal, with many small cysts of 2-4 mm in diameter, scattered within or arranged around the rim of the ovary, and there is increased stroma (the tissue between the cysts) within the ovary (Figure 5.4A). The uterus may be enlarged with a thickened endometrial lining (Figure 5.4B).

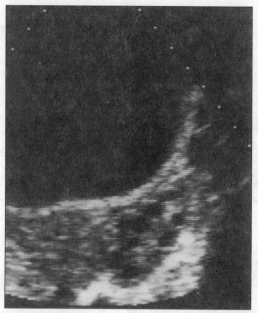

Figure 5.4A A polycystic ovary with multiple small cysts and highly echogenic stroma.

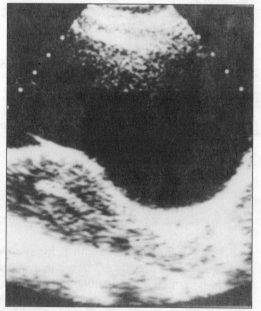

Figure 5.4B An enlarged uterus with thickened endometruim seen in a patient with polycystic ovarian syndrome.

The third type of picture is that seen in women with **multicystic ovaries**. In this case the ovaries may also be enlarged but contain cysts of 6-8 mm in diameter; there is no increase in the stromal tissue (Figure 5.5). Although there are fewer cysts than in the polycystic ovary their size is usually greater. The uterus is small and the endometrium thin.

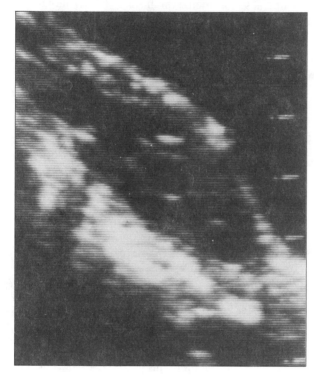

Figure 5.5 Multicystic ovary — notice that the cysts are larger than in the polycystic ovary and there is no increased stroma.

Multicystic ovaries occur normally in girls as they go through puberty. In adults, they may be seen in women who are beginning to recover from hypogonadotrophic hypogonadism, most typically in patients with anorexia nervosa who are regaining weight.

22. What is colour doppler ultrasound?

A very new ultrasound technique.

It measures the blood flow to and from the ovaries and the uterus. The degree of resistance to blood flow is shown by the shape of the doppler wave form (Figure 5.6A-B). It therefore provides a functional assessment of the receptivity of the uterus for implantation of the embryos.

Blood flowing away from the ultrasound scan probe shows up on the screen in blue while blood flowing towards it shows up in red. At the moment, doppler ultrasound is still at the research stage in infertility but initial results are encouraging.

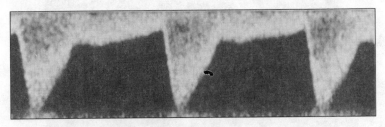

Figure 5.6A This doppler waveform indicates good blood flow.

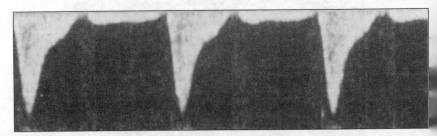

Figure 5.6B The doppler waveform in this photograph shows there is increased resistance to blood flow.

23. Can ultrasound scanning harm the eggs?
No.

There is no evidence at all that the doses of ultrasound used for infertility work causes any damage to the eggs.

24. How are changes in the cervical mucus used to detect the fertile period?
The cervical mucus is produced by glands in the cervical canal; it acts as a plug to prevent bacteria from getting into the uterus. The composition and

consistency of the cervical mucus changes during the menstrual cycle. During the initial part of the menstrual cycle it is scanty and thick. About 5 days before ovulation, the rise in the levels of oestrogen produced by the developing ovarian follicle causes the mucus to increase in amount and become more watery. Just before ovulation occurs, the mucus is very watery, slippery and stretchable, like raw egg-white.

After ovulation has occurred, mucus production almost completely stops within 24 hours and it then becomes thick and yellowish-white in colour.

25.   What is a post-coital test and how is it done?
This is one of the oldest tests used in infertility.

One or two days before ovulation occurs, you are advised to have intercourse the night before visiting the clinic. Most doctors consider that the test should be done between 6 and 12 hours after intercourse. While having a bath will not affect the test, a douche is inadvisable. In the clinic a speculum is inserted into the vagina and a small amount of mucus removed from the cervical canal. The procedure is painless. The mucus is then examined under a microscope and its quality noted. The number of sperm present is counted and their movement through the mucus recorded (Figure 5.7A-B).

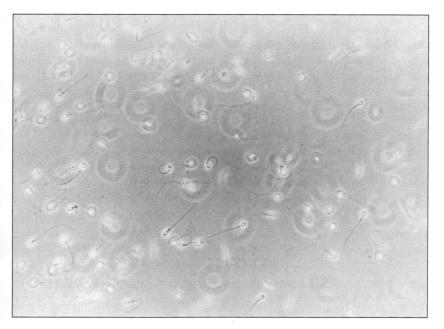

Figure 5.7A A good post-coital test showing many active sperm.

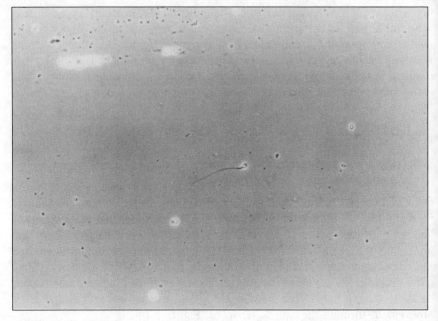

Figure 5.7B   A poor post-coital test showing almost complete absence of sperms.

26. What does a "good" post-coital test mean?

A good post-coital test (PCT) is one in which at least five sperm are seen in each microscopic field to be swimming actively in a straight line through the mucus.

A good PCT means that sperm are being produced, they are being deposited in the vagina and they are able to penetrate the cervical mucus to enter the uterus.

27. What are the causes of a "poor" post-coital test?

The most common reason for a poor PCT is wrong timing.

The test must be done when the mucus is very receptive and allows sperm to penetrate it. If the PCT is done too early or too late in the cycle the PCT will be abnormal because the mucus will be too thick. If by chance you had not ovulated in the particular menstrual cycle in which the test was done, oestrogen production would have been low and again the mucus very tenacious.

On the other hand, your partner may not have produced good quality or sufficient sperm. Sometimes there is a sexual problem and the sperm are not actually deposited within the vagina. Rarely there may be an abnormality of the cervix, for instance, a scarred cervix that cannot produce good mucus. Finally, there may be antibodies produced by the cervix which hinder the sperm motility (Chapter 13, question 7).

If there are conflicting results from several post coital tests, it is important to realise that the outlook for fertility is related to the *good* results, not the bad ones.

28.   Can infertility treatment cause sexual problems?
Yes, unfortunately it can.

While the couple's sexual relationship has previously been a spontaneous and intimate affair, they may find they are now expected to perform sex to order, having intercourse when the follicle is 18 mm on the ultrasound scan, when the basal body temperature dips, every other day from day 10 of the cycle and so on. When sex becomes essentially an exercise whose only function is to achieve pregnancy, the basis is laid for a great deal of tension. For example, it is not uncommon for couples to be unable to have sexual intercourse at the time specified for the post coital test.

It is important to know that many couples have this experience. It is one of those situations where discussions with an infertility counsellor may well be of help.

29.   How does the doctor check my fallopian tubes?
The methods are the Rubin's test, hysterosalpingogram and laparoscopic dye hydrotubation.

30.   Can my tubes be open and still not working?
The fallopian tubes play a vital part in fertilisation and the early development of the embryo. After ovulation, the egg does not passively drop into the fallopian tube but instead the fimbriae of the tube "search out" the egg and pick it up. Once the egg is inside the tube, its only source of nutrition is provided by the fluid secreted by the lining of the tube. Moreover, it moves along the tube towards the uterus by the movements of tiny hairs, called cilia, which line the fallopian tube as well as by the muscular contractions of the tube itself.

Therefore, even if the tube is open, it may not work properly. For example, it may be stuck down or kinked by adhesions so that the fimbriae cannot pick up the egg. Even after the egg has entered the tube, its nutrition and movement may be hampered if the lining of the tube is damaged.

31.   What is the Rubin's test?
A very old test, hardly ever used nowadays. It involved passing carbon dioxide

through the fallopian tubes and listening with a stethoscope for bubbling sounds as the gas escaped from the tubes.

32. Is the Rubin's test accurate?
No. It really should not be used these days.

33. Can an X-ray be taken to see if my tubes are blocked?
Yes, the test is called a **hysterosalpingogram** (HSG).

In this test a small amount of a special dye is injected into the uterus from below and is allowed to flow out of the tubes (Figure 5.8A). The dye shows up on the X-ray screen and if there is blockage of the fallopian tubes the dye will not flow through (Figure 5.8B). The amount of radiation it takes to perform this test is very small and is not harmful.

34. Do I need an anaesthetic for it?
No. But about 20 percent of women who have an HSG do experience some lower abdominal discomfort: fortunately this only lasts for a few minutes.

35. Do I have to stay in hospital for an HSG?
No. An HSG only takes a few minutes to perform and is an outpatient procedure.

36. What can an HSG tell?
A HSG tells us about the state of the uterine cavity (the hysterogram) as well as the inside of the fallopian tubes (the salpingogram).

If the tubes are blocked, the salpingogram will show the site of the blockage since dye cannot flow past the block. The HSG will also reveal any swelling of the tube (hydrosalpinx) which occurs because of tubal blockage (Figure 5.8B).

The hysterogram is useful to check the inside of the uterus, particularly in cases of recurrent miscarriage.

An HSG and laparoscopy are complementary investigations in the management of infertility. The HSG provides information about the inside condition of the uterus and fallopian tubes. The laparoscopy allows a direct view of the external surfaces of these organs.

37. What is a laparoscopy and how is it carried out?
A laparoscope is an instrument which allows the pelvic organs to be inspected under direct vision (Figure 5.9A-H). It looks like a telescope several inches long and is inserted into the abdomen. In the past the procedure was only used to diagnose pelvic problems. Nowadays it is also possible to perform corrective surgery through the laparoscope.

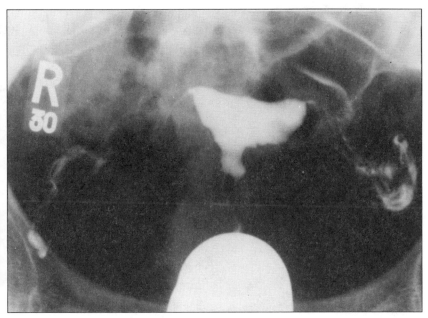

(a)   Dye can be seen spilling out of the fallopian tubes which are patent.

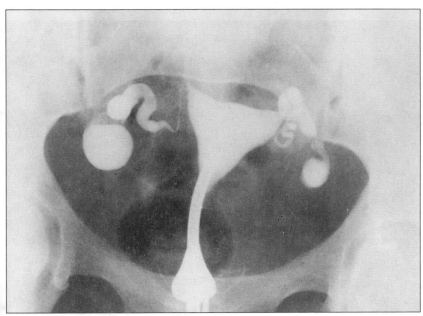

(b)   Hysterosalpingogram showing blocked fallopian tubes with hydrosalpinx

Figure 5.8   Normal and abnormal hysterosalpingograms.

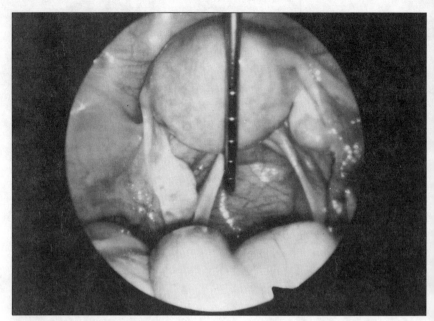

Figure 5.9A This shows a normal pelvis as seen on laparoscopy. There is a corpus luteum seen in the right ovary.

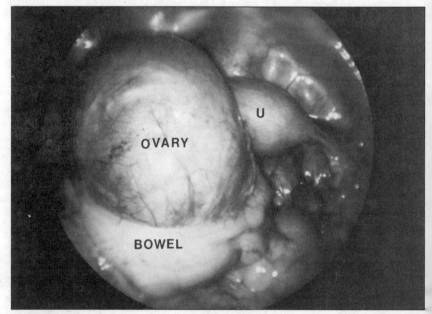

Figure 5.9B This photograph shows the uterus, ovary and bowel stuck together by adhesions.

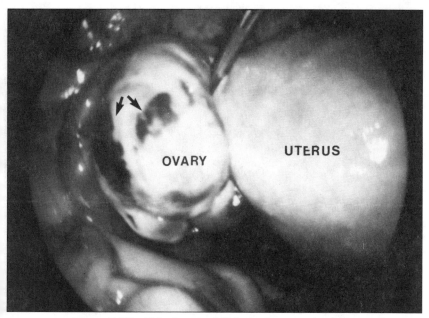

Figure 5.9C   This shows a follicle in the ovary (arrows).

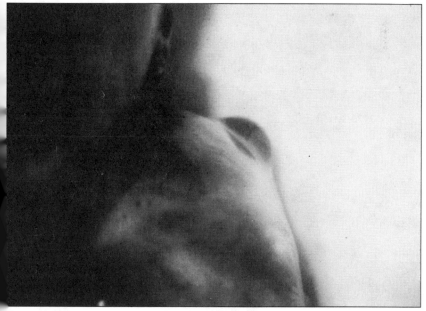

Figure 5.9D   This shows a follicle in the ovary on the verge of ovulating.

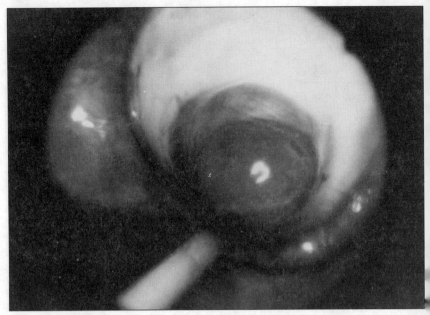

Figure 5.9E This shows a corpus luteum in the ovary.

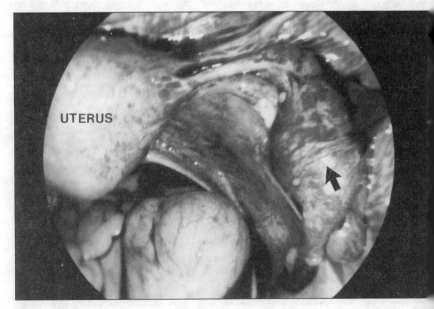

Figure 5.9F The arrow points to the end of the fallopian tube which has swollen to form a hydrosalpinx.

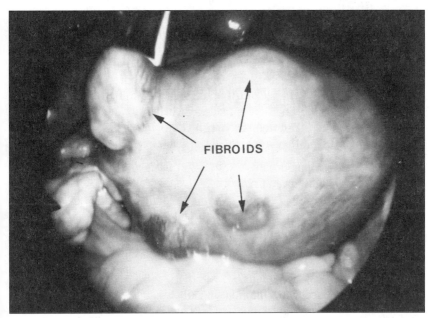

Figure 5.9G   Uterine fibroids seen on laparoscopy.

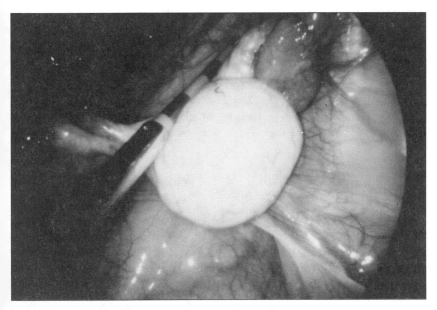

Figure 5.9H   A polycystic ovary as seen on laparoscopy.

The procedure is usually performed under general anaesthesia. A tiny incision is made just below the umbilicus (navel) and 3 litres or so of carbon dioxide are introduced to distend the abdominal cavity. This separates the bowel from the abdominal wall so that the laparoscope can be inserted safely. The laparoscope is then connected to a powerful light source which allows the surgeon to look inside the abdomen and directly examine the pelvic organs. A second, even smaller, incision is made just below the pubic hairline and a special pair of forceps inserted through it. Both incisions are so small that once they have healed they are virtually invisible.

A diagnostic laparoscopy usually takes 15-30 minutes. If infertility surgery is performed it may take several hours.

38. Do I need to stay in hospital for a laparoscopy?
It depends on the surgeon. Some will advise that you stay overnight in hospital while others treat the procedure as a day case.

39. Is a laparoscopy dangerous?
The risks of laparoscopy are minimal in skilled hands.

Most women feel rather bloated and uncomfortable for 24 hours or so after laparoscopy. Some feel a little pain around the shoulder for 1 or 2 days because of residual gas inside the abdomen which irritates the nerves (most of the gas is removed at the end of the operation).

About two per 1,000 women have some internal bleeding but this usually does not require further treatment. An equally small proportion of women have a puncture of the intestines which occurs when the laparoscope is inserted. In very rare cases, an immediate operation is necessary to repair the damage.

40. What does the surgeon look for at the time of laparoscopy?
The surgeon inspects the uterus, fallopian tubes, ovaries and the pelvic walls very carefully. Any scar tissue, adhesions and endometriosis is noted. The mobility of the ovaries and tubes can be assessed by using the pair of forceps inserted just below the pubic hairline. The ovaries are also inspected for signs of ovulation or the presence of cysts.

An assistant then injects a solution of a blue dye through the cervix into the uterus. It is then possible to see whether the dye enters the tubes, how rapidly it flows through them and whether it spills out of them easily. Finally, other abdominal organs such as the appendix, bowel, liver and gall bladder can be inspected through the laparoscope.

Most surgeons will remove a small piece of endometrium for examination as well. The sample of endometrium is sent to the pathologist for examination to see if there has been secretory changes caused by ovulation and whether there is any infection present, in particular, tuberculosis.

41. If I conceive in the cycle in which the laparoscopy is performed will it harm the baby?

If laparoscopy is performed in the second half of the menstrual cycle there is a very small possibility that you may have conceived in that cycle. The chance of the laparoscopy damaging the pregnancy is however very small. Nevertheless for your peace of mind, it is advisable to use some mechanical protection, such as a condom, during a cycle in which laparoscopy is going to be performed.

42.   What is hysteroscopy?

A hysteroscope is a telescopic instrument which allows the inside of the uterus to be inspected under direct vision (Figure 5.10).

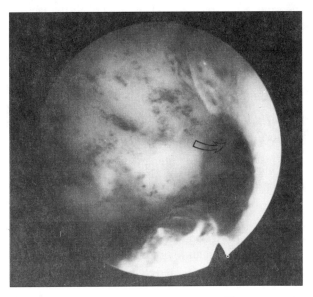

Figure 5.10 Hysteroscopic view of the uterine cavity. The arrow points to the entrance of the fallopian tube into the uterine cavity.

The patient is usually given a general anaesthetic (although some gynaecologists perform hysteroscopy as an out-patient procedure without a general anaesthetic). A little gas or fluid is introduced into the uterine cavity to open it up and the hysteroscope then inserted. It is attached to a powerful light source which allows the uterine cavity to be examined.

Hysteroscopy is particularly useful when problems inside the uterus are suspected — such as uterine adhesions (Asherman's syndrome), abnormalities of the uterine wall and a particular type of fibroid (submucous fibroid).

43. Why is a sperm test necessary?
Because an estimated one-third of infertility cases are caused by problems in the man and in another one-third, there may be problems in both partners. It is, therefore, essential to perform a sperm test as part of the work-up of every infertile couple.

44. What does a sperm test involve?
As the criteria for assessing sperm depend on a fixed period of abstinence, the man is asked to abstain from sex or masturbation for 3 days. He then has to produce a sample of semen by masturbation into a clean glass or plastic container. The sample of semen should be brought to the laboratory as soon as is practical, preferably within an hour of being produced. In cold weather the container should be kept in an inside pocket on the way to the laboratory.

45. What is checked in a sperm test?
In the usual semen analysis, the volume of the ejaculate, the acidity (pH) of the semen, the sperm density, percentage of motile sperm, the morphology (shape) of the sperm, and the number of white blood cells in the semen. A test is also usually done to detect sperm antibodies (the MAR test).

46. What is a normal sperm analysis?
The minimum criteria of a normal semen analysis are:

volume	: 1.5 ml
sperm density	: 20 million per ml
sperm motility	: at least 50 percent (1 hour after collection)
sperm morphology	: at least 60 percent normal forms
white blood cells	: no pus cells detected

These results are broadly indicative of the chances of pregnancy but they are not exact criteria. This means that, everything else being equal, a man with a sperm count that varies between 10-15 million/ml will probably take longer to get his partner pregnant than another man who has a sperm count of 60 million/ml.

47. Is one poor sperm test enough to diagnose male infertility?
No.

Sperm production can be depressed by a number of factors such as infection, drugs, heat, and cigarette smoking and the depressed sperm production can last anywhere from a few weeks to several years. Sperm counts can vary tremendously from one week to another, even in normal men. Male infertility should not, therefore, be diagnosed on the basis of a single semen analysis. It should only be diagnosed if the analyses are repeatedly abnormal.

48.   What is the purpose of surgical exploration of the testicles and testicular biopsy?
This is sometimes carried out to see if the testicle is producing sperm and whether there is a blockage of the ducts leading from them. If there is a blockage, the site of obstruction can also be detected. This investigation is not necessary in most cases and is rarely indicated.

49.   What is the hamster egg test?
This test is designed to assess the ability of sperm to penetrate eggs.

The sperm are specially prepared and mixed with hamster eggs that have had their outer coat stripped off. The percentage of hamster eggs that are penetrated can be used as a guide to the fertilising ability of the sperm. There is, however, doubt about the accuracy of this test because there are cases where the sperm are completely unable to penetrate the hamster eggs but are able to fertilise human eggs. For this reason, experts disagree about the value of the test.

6

HORMONE TESTS FOR INFERTILITY

1.   What hormone tests are done for infertility?

In women, the hormone tests commonly done for infertility are measurements of blood levels of follicle stimulating hormone (FSH), luteinising hormone (LH), oestradiol, prolactin, testosterone, and progesterone. Not all infertility patients require all these tests.

2.   Why are the levels of FSH, LH, oestradiol, prolactin, and testosterone measured?

These hormone concentrations are measured if the patient has irregular, infrequent or absent menstrual periods to try to determine the cause.

The first thing to say is that the results should be interpreted in the context of the patient's menstrual history, together with the results of all the other tests.

A high FSH and a low oestradiol concentration indicates primary ovarian failure (Chapter 7, question 6) while a high LH with a normal FSH level suggests polycystic ovary syndrome (Chapter 7, question 34). Subnormal LH and FSH, together with a low serum oestradiol concentration indicates hypogonadotrophic hypogonadism (Chapter 7, question 11). The prolactin level is measured to exclude hyperprolactinaemia (Chapter 7, question 19). A raised serum testosterone concentration supports a diagnosis of polycystic ovary syndrome; when it is very high (that is, in the range found in men) it suggests the presence of a rare type of tumour of the ovary or adrenal gland.

3.   What does the serum progesterone concentration indicate?   ˙

Progesterone is the hormone produced by the corpus luteum after ovulation has occurred. It is measured to see if the patient has ovulated, either spontaneously or in response to treatment. It is crucial for correct interpretation to measure it 1 week after (anticipated) ovulation, that is, on or about day 21 of a 28-day cycle.

A serum progesterone concentration of 30 nmol/L (10ng/ml) or higher on day 21 of a 28-day cycle suggests the patient has ovulated.

4.   What hormone test kits can be used to predict ovulation?
Just before ovulation occurs, the pituitary gland releases the mid-cycle surge of LH which can be detected as a brief peak of LH in blood or urine about 24-36 hours before ovulation.

There are now a number of test kits available which can be used to detect the LH surge. Using such kits, the woman can test her urine each day around the time the LH surge is expected. A colour reaction indicates that ovulation is about to occur.

Examples of some kits that are commercially available are Ovustick, Ovuqick, First Response, Q Test, OvuGen, Fortel, Clearplan, Night Day and Answer.

5.   Why do I need several blood tests during induction of ovulation?
Several reasons, depending on what exactly the doctor is trying to achieve:

a)   To be as sure as possible that you have indeed ovulated — a progesterone measurement on day 21 (that is, during the luteal phase).

b)   To be as sure as possible that only one follicle is developing in response to ovarian stimulation — several measurements of oestradiol in the follicular phase of the cycle, say, on days 8, 10 and 12. These measurements can be made on samples of blood or urine.

   In some fertility clinics ultrasound assessment of the ovarian follicles and the uterus (the endometrium grows in response to oestrogen secretion by the follicle) is used instead of, or as well as, oestrogen measurements.

c)   To be sure that LH concentrations are not inappropriately high in patients with polycystic ovary syndrome — a measurement of the serum LH concentration in the follicular phase (for example, on day 8).

These tests usually need to be done in at least one cycle. If the LH concentration is satisfactory, no more LH measurements are necessary. If a simple method of ovarian stimulation (like clomiphene or tamoxifen) is being used then oestradiol measurements will not be needed but if hMG is being used, such measurements are obligatory.

6.   Are hormone tests helpful in men?
Not so often as in women.

If there is a very low sperm count, less than 5 million/ml, then the level of FSH and testosterone should be measured. If the FSH is high it means that the testes have failed to respond to the appropriate hormonal stimulation. This implies that the process of sperm production is so impaired that no treatment will be of any benefit.

On the other hand, a normal serum FSH concentration in a man with azoospermia suggests the cause is a blockage that is preventing the sperm from reaching the ejaculate (for example, as occurs after a vasectomy). Such cases need evaluation by a surgeon specialising in male infertility to determine whether the blockage can be relieved surgically.

If the level of FSH is very low, a pituitary tumour should be considered. An X-ray of the skull is done and the prolactin level checked. If the serum prolactin concentration is high treatment can then be given in the form of bromocriptine tablets (Chapter 7, question 21). This treatment will put the hormone disturbance right and also cause the pituitary tumour to shrink.

The level of testosterone is checked because if it is low then hormone replacement should be given. This will not improve the sperm count but is important as lowered levels of testosterone may lead to weakness, lethargy, reduced hair growth on the body, decreased libido and impotence.

7

ANOVULATION

1. What are the causes of anovulation?
Anything that disconnects the various links between the hypothalamus, pituitary gland and ovaries (Chapter 1, question 4) can make the reproductive system falter and cause anovulation.

If there is damage directly to the hypothalamus or pituitary gland, or if the ovary does not respond to the pituitary hormones, then there will be failure of ovulation. Occasionally, ovulatory failure occurs because of over or underactivity of another gland such as the thyroid or adrenals.

Almost all women occasionally miss a few periods. A common example would be a girl preparing for her examinations. The stress she experiences may cause her not to ovulate. Such temporary disruption of ovulation, however, does not cause infertility.

2. If I have no periods does it mean I am not ovulating?
Yes, usually it does.

When a woman has no periods for 6 months or more, she is said to have **amenorrhoea**. A woman with amenorrhoea is almost certainly not ovulating. There is a condition, however, in which amenorrhoea is caused by damage to the endometrial lining of the uterus which is then incapable of responding to oestrogen (Ashermann's syndrome) but it is very rare.

3. If I have infrequent or irregular periods does it mean I'm not ovulating?
You may either not be ovulating or ovulating less frequently than normally.

When a woman has periods once every 6 weeks to 6 months she is said to have **oligomenorrhoea**. Most women with infrequent or irregular periods are either not ovulating or are ovulating irregularly. In either case, the lower rate of ovulation means that the chances of getting pregnant are reduced.

For example, if ovulation occurs only five times in a year instead of the usual thirteen times, the chance of getting pregnant during that year falls to 5/13, that is, 38 percent, of what it might have been. Another way of looking at it is that, on average, it would take a woman having five ovulations a year more than twice as long to conceive than if she were having a regular 28-day cycle. Moreover, having irregular cycles makes it difficult to be sure when ovulation does occur. That also contributes to the problem because it is likely that some ovulations will then be "missed".

4. I am 25 years old and have never had a period without hormone treatment. Can I possibly conceive?
Yes, the chances are good.

A woman who has never had a period spontaneously is said to have **primary amenorrhoea**.

If you have primary amenorrhoea the chance of conception depends entirely on the cause. Table 7.1 shows you the causes in 90 consecutive cases we have seen in our clinics over the last few years.

Table 7.1 Causes of primary amenorrhoea.

Premature (primary) ovarian failure .... (premature menopause)	36 percent
Hypogonadotrophic hypogonadism	34 percent
Polycystic ovary syndrome	17 percent
Hypopituitarism	4 percent
Hyperprolactinaemia	3 percent
Weight related amenorrhoea	2 percent
Congenital abnormalities	4 percent

Contrary to popular belief, in most cases of amenorrhoea the chances of having a child are very high, provided the correct treatment is given.

5. I am 30 years old and my periods were regular until 2 years ago when they stopped. What are the likely causes?
When periods stop after having been established, we use the term **secondary amenorrhoea**.

In Table 7.2 you can see the causes of secondary amenorrhoea in 400 consecutive cases we have seen in our clinics.

Table 7.2 Causes of secondary amenorrhoea.

Polycystic ovary syndrome	30 percent
Premature ovarian failure	29 percent
Weight related amenorrhoea	19 percent
Hyperprolactinaemia	14 percent
(including prolactinoma)	
Exercise related amenorrhoea	2 percent
Hypopituitarism	2 percent
Miscellaneous	4 percent

6. What do you mean by premature menopause?

A menopause is defined as being premature if it occurs before the age of 40.

It is diagnosed when a woman whose periods have stopped before she is 40 years old is found on blood tests to have high FSH (and LH) and low oestradiol levels. The ultrasound shows small ovaries, with a small uterus and thin endometrium. The alternative term for this condition is **premature ovarian failure**.

It is the most serious cause of amenorrhoea because it means there is something wrong with the ovaries themselves. The astonishing thing is that premature menopause can occur at any age. It may therefore present as primary (see Table 7.1) or as secondary amenorrhoea (see Table 7.2).

7. What causes premature ovarian failure (premature menopause)?

There are a number of causes.

First, the woman might have been born with fewer eggs than normal. That is what happens in patients with **Turner's syndrome**, a condition in which the one of the X chromosomes is missing. Patients with Turner's syndrome are usually of short stature and have delay in the onset of puberty. They typically (but not inevitably) present with primary amenorrhoea. The diagnosis is confirmed by a blood test in which the chromosomes are specifically identified (**karyotype**).

Second, the ovaries may have been damaged by infection (for example, mumps), by surgery or by medications used in the treatment of certain cancers. Like irradiation of the ovaries, the drugs nearly always damage the ovaries when they are used in the doses necessary for treating these conditions. Sometimes these medications are also required for non-malignant conditions, such as severe inflamation of the blood vessels (vasculitis). Examples of these drugs are cyclophosphamide, busulphan and chlorambucil.

Third, there is evidence that as many as half the cases are caused by **autoimmunity**. The reason we do not get a second attack of measles, for example, is that we develop immunity (resistance) to the virus and our cells destroy it the next time it tries to get into our bodies. Some people have an immune defense system that is so sensitive that it fires off too easily and fails to distinguish between their own tissues and the foreign invader (the virus). For some reason, hormone secreting glands such as the thyroid and the ovary are particularly vulnerable to this condition.

Finally, there are many cases of premature ovarian failure in which we simply do not know why the rate of removal of eggs and follicles from the ovaries is so much faster than normal (Chapter 1, question 3). As usual, these cases are called "idiopathic".

8. Is there any fertility treatment for premature ovarian failure?

There is no effective treatment as long as the amenorrhoea, subnormal oestrogen and high FSH levels remain. Occasionally the condition gets better spontaneously but we know of no reliable way to predict which cases will improve. Certainly there is no treatment that has been proven to make the ovulation cycle return.

9. Is there any chance then for a woman who has premature ovarian failure to get pregnant?

It is most unlikely, unless she has eggs donated to her by another woman (ovum donation — Chapter 11, question 44).

10. My doctor tells me that I have had a premature menopause. Do I need hormone treatment?

Yes, you do.

We know that women who have premature ovarian failure are at risk from all the problems associated with lack of oestrogen, including a high risk of osteoporosis (that is, brittle bones in the spine, wrist and hips that tend to fracture easily).

For this reason we advise treatment with oestrogen. If you take oestrogen it is necessary to take progesterone as well to ensure the uterus is not over-stimulated. The simplest way to do that these days is to take a combined oestrogen and progestogen containing birth control pill. It is taken cyclically for 3 weeks and then stopped for 1 week, during which a period occurs. Special care is obviously needed in a youngster with primary amenorrhoea in whom oestrogen replacement should be started with very low doses.

If you are keen to have a child (although, we emphasise the chances without ovum donation are very slim), the doctor may advise you to stop the hormones for 2 months or so each year. If you continue to have menstrual periods after the hormone pills have been stopped and the level of FSH returns to normal, you may be one of those lucky individuals who have a spontaneous return of ovarian function. You should not, however, count on this happening because only a small proportion of women who have premature menopause recover spontaneously.

11. What is hypogonadotrophic hypogonadism?

This is a condition in which the pituitary gland does not secrete the gonadotrophins (LH and FSH) in sufficient amounts to stimulate the gonad (the ovary).

In some cases the cause is a congenital absence of LHRH, the hypothalamic (brain) hormone that is normally released in pulses and stimulates the pituitary to secrete LH and FSH. If the condition is congenital the person does not go through puberty and presents to the doctor as a case of primary amenorrhoea.

Sometimes hypogonadotrophic hypogonadism occurs in association with impaired secretion of other pituitary hormones. It is then part of a more generalised hypopituitarism (question 12).

The most common form of hypogonadotrophic hypogonadism is that caused by subnormal nutrition (weight related amenorrhoea, question 13). Whatever the cause, however, the hormonal findings are of subnormal blood concentrations of LH, FSH and oestradiol, associated with the ultrasound findings of small ovaries and a small uterus.

The fertility outlook for patients with hypogonadotrophic hypogonadism is excellent: if the condition has been caused by a reduction in LHRH release it is treated with pulsatile LHRH therapy. If it is the result of pituitary failure it is treated with hMG injections (Chapter 8, question 14). The only cases needing a different form of treatment are when the cause is a prolactinoma, in which case the treatment is with bromocriptine (question 24) and when the cause is subnormal weight, in which case regaining weight is usually sufficient to correct the amenorrhoea and infertility (question 15).

12. What is hypopituitarism?

Hypopituitarism means that the pituitary gland is secreting its hormones in insufficient amounts, if at all.

If the deficiency is entirely in the secretion of LH and FSH, it is called hypogonadotrophic hypogonadism and the patient presents with amenorrhoea; if the onset is in childhood there will also be delay in the onset of puberty. If the condition is associated with other hormone deficiencies, the child may fail to grow (growth hormone deficiency) or have evidence of thyroid or adrenal failure.

Hypopituitarism is sometimes caused by a pituitary tumour (question 21) but often the cause is never diagnosed. Sometimes the cause is a disturbance of the hypothalamus, rather than the pituitary itself.

13. What is weight related amenorrhoea?
It is well known that menstrual periods stop in women who lose weight because of anorexia nervosa and return when weight is regained.

Recent work has shown that in these patients it is primarily the fall in weight that causes the amenorrhoea. Moreover, it has been found that any cause of subnutrition may be associated with amenorrhoea if the loss of weight is sufficient. It does not seem to matter whether the cause is lack of available food (as in famines) or a reluctance to eat food that is available (as in anorexia nervosa) or a failure to absorb food (as in malabsorption syndromes). Furthermore, even when the intake of food is normal, amenorrhoea may develop if the weight falls because the calories are used up by high intensity athletics (as in runners, gymnasts and ballet dancers) or by an overactive metabolism (as in hyperthyroidism).

14. Is there a critical weight at which periods stop?
There is no single normal (or abnormal) weight for all women, after all, our weight normally varies with age and with our build. There is, however, a range of normality. An easy way to determine the appropriate weight for one's height is to calculate the body mass index (BMI).

The formula is BMI = weight (in kgs) ÷ height^2 (in metres).

Normally the BMI lies between 20 and 25. You can see the relationship between height and weight in Figure 7.1.

To calculate your own BMI the first thing to do is to convert your height and weight to their metric equivalents. For weight, since there are 2.2 lbs per kg, you convert the stones to pounds and then divide by 2.2. Thus for a woman whose weight is 7 stone 4 lbs, the weight in kgs is = 7 x 14 + 4 lbs = 102 lbs ÷ 2.2 = 46.36 kgs.

For height, since there are 2.5 cm per inch, you convert the feet to inches and multiply by 2.5. To get the figure in metres you divide by 100. Thus for a woman 5 foot 4 inches tall, her height in metres is 64 inches x 2.5 ÷ 100 = 1.6 metres.

So the body mass index is 46.36 ÷ 1.6^2 = 18.1.

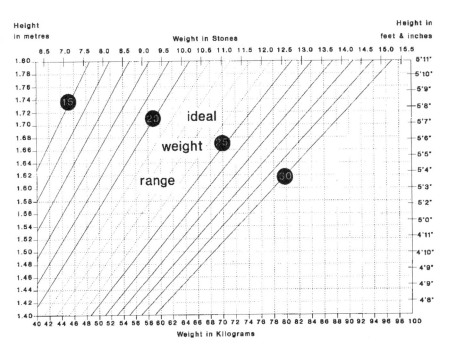

Figure 7.1 Body Mass Index calculation chart. The diagonal lines give the BMI (the figures in the dark circles) for any combination of height and weight.

In most women the menstrual period stops when the BMI falls below 19 and resumes when the weight comes up to give a BMI of 20.

15. I weigh 7 stones 4 lbs and am 5 foot 4 inches tall. My doctor has asked me to put on weight to regain my period. How do I calculate the amount of weight I need to regain?
First rearrange the formula so that

BMI = weight ÷ height² becomes weight = height² x BMI

Since your height is 5 foot 4 inches (= 64 inches x 2.5 ÷ 100 = 1.6 metres) and the normal BMI is 20-25, your minimum required weight is therefore 1.6m² x 20 = 51.2 kgs.

The difference between your actual weight (46.36 kgs) and the weight that will give you a BMI of 20 (51.2 kgs) is the amount you need to put on, that is, 4.84 kgs (x 2.2 = 10.6 lbs).

16. How much do I have to eat to be able to put on that amount of weight?
Again this involves some arithmetic.

One pound of fat is equivalent to about 3,500 calories. What this means is that if you eat 3,500 calories worth of food more than you are eating at present you will put on a pound in weight. The only decision now is how fast to do it.

Imagine you decide to put on a pound a week (actually this is for argument only — it would be too fast and we would not recommend doing it so quickly). That would mean eating 3,500 calories more per week, which is 3,500 ÷ 7 (= 500) calories per day or 500 ÷ 3 (= 166) calories more per meal. As we said, this is an unrealistically fast rate and it would be more appropriate for you to increase your weight by a pound a fortnight. To put on a pound every two weeks you would have to eat 166 ÷ 2 calories more at every meal and that would be a reasonable change to make to your diet.

Since you need to increase your weight by 10.6 lbs, that should take just over 5 months if you can stick to this diet.

So far as which food to eat, it is best to get a book on the caloric value of different foods. The crucial thing is to increase your overall intake and so long as you have a balanced diet, the particular foods do not matter too much.

17. This is all very well but you do not seem to understand the difficulty I have in putting on weight.
We do appreciate how difficult it can be and understand that the reasons for being underweight are often very profound. But the problem is that nature has tied nutrition and reproduction very tightly together - some of the reasons are described in Chapter 8, question 1.

In the United Kingdom many people with eating difficulties find they can get help from organisations like

> The Eating Disorders Association, Sackville Place
> 44-48 Magdelen Street, Norwich
> Norfolk NR3 IJE
> (telephone number 0603-621414)

but we hope that you will also discuss these problems with your own doctor.

18. I have heard that exercise can cause amenorrhoea. Can you tell me something about this?
In recent years it has become clear that women who compete at a high level in certain sports may stop menstruating and the term "exercise related amenorrhoea" has been coined.

There are three important points about this condition. First, for exercise to result in amenorrhoea it has to be of high intensity, as, for example, in sportswomen training for competitive athletics. Playing tennis twice a week or jogging round the park a few times will not cause amenorrhoea. Second, only certain sports seem to be associated with amenorrhoea, namely those that lead to a fall in body fat content. Thus gymnasts, runners, athletes and ballet dancers are vulnerable to amenorrhoea but swimmers, who retain their fat for buoyancy, are not. Third, exercise related amenorrhoea is temporary and menstrual cycles should return when the competitive season is over.

19.   My periods have stopped and my doctor has told me that it is because my prolactin level is very high. Can you please explain?
Prolactin is the hormone produced by the pituitary gland that is responsible for the production of milk and the amenorrhoea that women experience after childbirth. It is normally only secreted in large amounts during pregnancy and when the baby suckles at the breast. Sometimes it can be secreted in large amounts at inappropriate times - in this situation too it stops the periods but, because the breasts have not been stimulated by the high oestrogen levels of pregnancy, they do not produce much milk.

Oversecretion of prolactin **(hyperprolactinaemia)** prevents the intermittent release of LHRH from the hypothalamus (Chapter 1, question 4). Without this LHRH signal, the pituitary gland does not secrete FSH and LH in the normal way. There is, therefore, no follicular development, little oestrogen made, no ovulation and no periods.

20.   What is galactorrhoea? Is it a reliable sign of a raised prolactin level?
Galactorrhoea means inappropriate milk secretion — that is, not associated with recent childbirth.

There are two types — galactorrhoea that only occurs when you (or the doctor) express the milk from the nipples; medically unimportant, the best treatment is to stop looking for it.

On the other hand, galactorrhoea that is spontaneous (that is, it leaks from the breast without being expressed) usually signifies hyperprolactinaemia, particularly if it is associated with amenorrhoea. However, since galactorrhoea occurs in only a third of women with hyperprolactinaemia and amenorrhoea, measurement of blood concentrations of prolactin remains the cornerstone of diagnosis.

It is important to know that galactorrhoea is not a sign of breast cancer. Women with galactorrhoea and with hyperprolactinaemia do not have an increased risk of breast cancer.

21. What causes prolactin levels to be high (hyperprolactinaemia)?
There are five causes.

The first is taking certain drugs — both narcotics like heroin and medications such as certain tranquilliser (phenothiazines) and indigestion remedies, like metoclopramide (Maxolon). Your doctor will know straight away if you are being prescribed one of these medications.

The second is an underactive thyroid gland (**hypothyroidism**). This is simple to diagnose with blood tests, which are in fact usually done whenever the prolactin concentration is measured. Hypothyroidism and any associated hyperprolactinaemia is easily treated with thyroid hormone tablets.

The third is a benign prolactin-secreting tumour of the pituitary gland (**prolactinoma**).

We repeat — a prolactinoma is a **benign** tumour of the pituitary gland. It is **not** a brain tumour and **not** cancer. A malignant (cancerous) prolactinoma has never been recorded in the medical literature. It is important to realise that the word "tumour" is being used here in the Latin sense of "swelling".

About half the cases of hyperprolactinaemia are caused by prolactinomas. The exact figure depends on how sensitive the method of diagnosis is; if you rely on ordinary X-rays the figure is much lower than when modern CT scans are done.

Prolactinomas are treated with bromocriptine tablets (question 29).

The fourth is a benign non-prolactin secreting pituitary tumour. Again we emphasise that this is benign and not a brain tumour. It raises the prolactin level by pressing on the hypothalamus. It does not respond to treatment with bromocriptine and is usually removed surgically or treated by X-rays.

The fifth is idiopathic — which is doctor-speak for "we do not know the cause". Probably many of these cases have tiny prolactinomas that cannot be seen even with the most sensitive methods. These cases respond well to treatment with bromocriptine.

22. What tests are done to investigate someone with hyperprolactinaemia (raised prolactin levels)?
The first thing the doctor will do is confirm that the prolactin level is indeed raised by repeating the test. If a particular medication is suspected as the cause, an alternative treatment will be recommended instead. The thyroid hormone levels will be checked and, if low, thyroid hormone tablets prescribed.

A simple X-ray of the skull will be taken and if the pituitary region is enlarged or the level of prolactin is very high, a special X-ray called a CT scan will be performed to see if a pituitary tumour is present. It is likely that an even more sensitive method — the MRI scan — will soon be used for investigating pituitary disorders.

23. What is the treatment for a patient with a raised prolactin level not caused by medication, thyroid disease or a pituitary tumour?
Bromocriptine tablets.

This drug belongs to a group called dopamine agonists. Several of them are now available but bromocriptine is the best known. It has been in use for about 15 years so there is a lot of experience with it.

24. How is bromocriptine taken?
With meals, because it can cause nausea if you take it on an empty stomach. At the beginning of treatment it may cause giddiness when you stand up so you normally start with a small dose (half a tablet — 1.25 mgs) taken at bedtime together with some food.

Provided there are no side effects, after 2-3 days the dose is increased to one tablet (2.5 mgs) at night with food. After a week or so, you can then take one tablet at night and one in the day time, again as part of a meal. A few days later the dose is raised to three tablets a day.

After 4-6 weeks of treatment the blood test is repeated. It is sensible to measure progesterone as well on this sample: the plan is for the prolactin to have fallen into the normal range and the progesterone to have risen, to indicate that ovulation has occurred. If this has not happened the dose of bromocriptine is increased.

We usually find that as soon as the menstrual cycle has become re-established the dose can be reduced — it seems that the dose needed to reverse hyperprolactinaemia is larger than the dose needed to keep the prolactin level in the normal range.

25. How effective is bromocriptine in treating hyperprolactinaemia?
Very.

It usually reduces prolactin levels to normal in a few weeks. Most remarkably, it also causes prolactinomas to shrink.

In the treatment of infertility, once the prolactin levels return to normal, ovulatory menstrual cycles return and the chances of getting pregnant become the same as that of a normal woman.

26. What are the side effects of bromocriptine?

The immediate side effects are nausea and vomiting if the drug is taken on an empty stomach and giddiness, which is caused by a tendency of the blood pressure to fall when standing up suddenly. These side effects are usually transient and can be avoided by following the advice given in the answer to question 24.

During long term treatment some women complain of a stuffy nose and constipation. The latter can usually be overcome by increasing the amount of bran in the diet. Occasionally Raynaud's syndrome (cold sensitivity of the hands) is made worse. Gastric bleeding has rarely been recorded.

27. Do all patients with raised prolactin levels need treatment?

Most of them do.

The reason is that even if fertility is not the problem, there are other adverse effects of hyperprolactinaemia.

Because the pulsatile release of LHRH is so severely impaired, women with this condition make very little oestrogen. This has two major effects. The first is that the vagina becomes oestrogen deficient so most women with hyperprolactinaemia find they suffer from dryness and discomfort during intercourse. The second is that oestrogen deficiency can harm other parts of the body — for instance, the bones, which may develop osteoporosis (brittleness). Finally, for reasons that we do not really understand, hyperprolactinaemia impairs libido, so both women and men with this condition usually lose interest in sex.

All of these problems get better when prolactin levels return to normal.

28. What is a prolactinoma?

A prolactinoma is a benign tumour of the pituitary gland that secretes prolactin.

It is called a **microadenoma** (microprolactinoma) if it is less than 1 cm and a **macroadenoma** (macroprolactinoma) if it is larger than 1 cm in diameter. Most prolactinomas do not seem to increase in size over the years and so, apart from oversecretion of prolactin, cause no problems at all. In about 10 percent of cases, a macroprolactinoma extends upwards, out of the pituitary fossa (suprasellar extension — Figure 7.2A). Patients with suprasellar extension need treatment (usually with bromocriptine) to ensure the prolactinoma does not press on the nerves.

29. What are the different treatments available for a prolactinoma?

There are three types of treatment, namely, medical treatment with bromocriptine, surgery or radiotherapy.

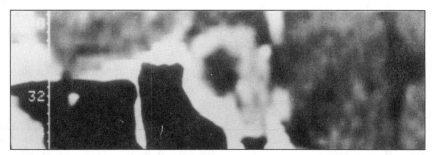

Figure 7.2A CT scan of the pituitary fossa showing a large prolactin secreting tumour (macroadenoma).

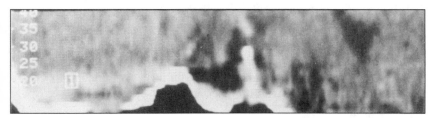

Figure 7.2B CT scan of the pituitary fossa in the same patient after bromocriptine therapy. The tumour has regressed.

More than 90 percent of prolactinomas shrink on treatment with bromocriptine (Figure 7.2B). Even very large tumours respond. In fact, bromocriptine is so effective that if the prolactin level returns to normal but the tumour does not shrink, the presence of a non-prolactin secreting pituitary tumour, which has raised prolactin levels by compressing the hypothalamus (question 21), should be suspected.

30. Can you tell me something about surgery and radiotherapy for prolactinomas?

There have been major advances in pituitary surgery in the last few years. What was really a big operation has been greatly simplified because, nowadays, the surgeon can operate through the nose (the **transphenoidal** approach). A microscope and instruments as fine as jeweller's tools are used. This means there is no scar and the patient is in hospital for only about a week. The transphenoidal approach has greatly reduced the incidence of surgical complications.

Despite these advances, we advise surgery only for patients who are resistant to bromocriptine (rare) or who get persistent side effects from it.

About 6 weeks after the operation, the patient returns to hospital for tests to ensure that the prolactin level has returned to normal and that the remainder of the pituitary hormones are satisfactory.

Radiotherapy is rarely needed for prolactinomas but is quite often used after surgery for non-prolactin secreting pituitary tumours. It involves having treatments spaced over 5-6 weeks on a special piece of equipment called a linear accelerator.

31. What are the arguments for medical treatments compared with surgical ones?

The main problem with medical treatment is that often the tablets have to be taken long term because once they are stopped the raised prolactin level may return and the menstrual periods disappear.

In the case of small tumours (microadenomas), most doctors nowadays advise medical treatment. With regard to large tumours (macroadenomas), some doctors feel that surgery is preferable because if it works, the patient has a permanent cure and does not require long term medication. In our experience, additional treatment with bromocriptine is so often required as to make this advantage illusory.

32. Are there any special precautions for a patient with a prolactinoma who wants to get pregnant?

Yes.

The main worry used to be that the prolactinoma might enlarge during pregnancy. The risk with microadenomas is very small indeed and even with macroadenomas is much lower than previously thought.

We therefore advise medical treatment initially for all prolactinoma patients. In patients with a macroprolactinoma, pregnancy should be avoided until a repeat CT scan has shown that the tumour has shrunk adequately. The repeat CT scan is done 3 months after starting treatment. In the small minority of cases where shrinkage has been insufficient, we then advise surgery. Using this approach, pregnancy in prolactinoma cases is very safe and no special treatment during pregnancy is required.

Once the patient is pregnant, treatment with bromocriptine should be stopped. This advice is given on the general principle that no drugs that are not definitely required should be taken during pregnancy. The patient is closely followed-up during pregnancy and if there is evidence of tumour expansion (rarely) treatment with bromocriptine can be safely re-introduced.

Careful follow-up studies of children born to women taking bromocriptine have shown no additional risk of congenital abnormalities associated with this drug.

33. What are polycystic ovaries?

The term polycystic ovaries refers to a particular appearance of the ovaries. Polycystic ovaries are usually larger than normal, with a smooth outer covering that is thicker than normal. The surface of the ovary is covered with many tiny cysts and there is increased tissue (stroma) between the cysts. The increase in stroma is just as important as the presence of the cysts. Incidently these cysts are harmless - they are not the type that causes pain and have nothing to do with cancer.

Figure 5.4A and 5.9H show the appearance of polycystic ovaries on pelvic ultrasonography and at laparoscopy.

34. What is the difference between polycystic ovaries, polycystic ovary disease and polycystic ovary syndrome?

"Polycystic ovaries" refers to the appearance of the ovaries, as described above and as found at laparoscopy or on an ultrasound scan.

Polycystic ovary syndrome (PCOS) is diagnosed when a patient with polycystic ovaries complains of the following:

a)   a menstrual disturbance — usually oligomenorrhoea, sometimes amenorrhoea, occasionally periods that are too frequent;

b)   the symptoms of too much testosterone - acne, greasy skin and unwanted hair;

c)   obesity.

Polycystic ovary disease is a misnomer — this is a technical point of medical classification but the condition we are talking about is a syndrome, not a disease.

As a result of being able to detect polycystic ovaries by ultrasound (a great advance, by the way, previously it was only possible at laparoscopy), we now know that polycystic ovaries are commonly seen even in perfectly healthy women. One study has reported their presence in more than 20 percent of young women who volunteered to have a scan. The appearance of polycystic ovaries is in itself nothing to worry about — polycystic ovaries only become a problem when they are associated with the symptoms described above.

35. What causes polycystic ovary syndrome?

Our research has shown that polycystic ovaries usually run in families. When we scan the daughters of our patients if they are old enough, or their mothers if they are young enough, or their sisters if they are available, we nearly always find they have polycystic ovaries as well. Sometimes we have even seen the appearance in girls before puberty. For these reasons we think the ovarian condition is inherited and probably present from a very young age.

What causes a woman with polycystic ovaries to develop polycystic ovary syndrome is one of the most important areas of present research in this area. We only know some of the factors.

The most important seems to be something to do with putting on weight. There is evidence that the ovary can be stimulated by insulin and that the polycystic ovary is particularly sensitive to this hormone. Insulin is secreted by the pancreas every time we eat and in overweight people more insulin is released for the same amount of food than in slim people. So if a woman happens to be born with polycystic ovaries, putting on weight makes the ovarian condition worse. There is also some evidence that women who have polycystic ovary syndrome tend to be overweight anyway so there is a vicious circle that develops here. But the only way to deal with it is to break the circle by loosing weight. This explanation cannot account for all cases — because only about a third to half of the patients with polycystic ovary syndrome are overweight. Research is actively seeking an explanation for the other cases.

36. What is the treatment for polycystic ovary syndrome?
It depends on what the patient is complaining of.

In this book we shall assume that the main complaint is infertility. The first thing to do is to try to get the overweight patient to lose weight because without doing that the chances of responding to treatment are very poor. In fact, losing weight by itself is often enough to put things right.

The next thing to do is to check that the serum LH concentration during the follicular phase is normal. For a woman having menstrual cycles this means having the blood test on day 7 to day 9 of the cycle. If menstrual cycles are very infrequent, then anytime except during the 10 days before a period is satisfactory. That means having the blood test and then waiting to be sure a period does not occur in the next 10 days before trying to interpret it.

If the serum LH level is raised, any form of treatment used to induce ovulation should also aim to reduce it because oversecretion of this hormone can impair fertility and also cause miscarriage, even in women who are ovulating normally. The particular LH concentration that is critical depends on the exact method of measurement and that is something you have to check with your doctor. For women with a high LH level we advise treatment with tamoxifen (Chapter 8, question 12) rather than clomiphene (Chapter 8, question 2). If that is successful, that is, it induces ovulation, as shown by either ultrasound scans or serum progesterone measurements or both, and keeps the follicular phase LH in the normal range, then treatment with that drug is appropriate and is continued.

If treatment with tamoxifen is unsuccessful and the patient is slim we advise treatment by **ovarian diathermy** (Chapter 8, question 50). This operation is done under general anaesthetia through the laparoscope and only involves being in hospital for one night. Again it is vital that blood tests are done to check that the LH level comes down to normal and that the cycle that emerges is ovulatory.

If the operation cannot be done because the patient is overweight, then treatment becomes a bit more complicated. An analogue of LHRH is first given to lower the LH concentrations and then the ovaries are stimulated by gonadotrophins. This treatment is described on page 93 .

Finally, if the patient is not ovulating and the serum LH concentration is not raised, treatment with clomiphene or tamoxifen is given; if there is no response, or the response is inadequate, ovulation is induced with pulsatile LHRH therapy (Chapter 8, question 25) or gonadotrophin injections (Chapter 8, question 15).

37. What is an inadequate luteal phase?

An inadequate luteal phase is one where there is ovulation but the corpus luteum does not produce an adequate amount of progesterone. It is diagnosed either by taking a small piece of endometrium (endometrial biopsy) for examination or by measuring the levels of progesterone serially in the second half of the menstrual cycle. An allied condition is a "short" luteal phase, in which the interval between ovulation and menstruation is shortened to less than 10 days. It is probably a more severe form of "inadequate" luteal phase. In both conditions the likelihood of an embryo implanting may be reduced.

38. What is the treatment for an inadequate luteal phase?

The treatment of an inadequate luteal phase depends on the cause. If it occurs because the follicle does not grow well, clomiphene citrate (Chapter 8, question 2) is often given to stimulate follicular growth. If the follicles grow normally and adequate amounts of oestrogen are produced, intermittent injections of hCG or progesterone tablets or suppositories are sometimes prescribed to support the corpus luteum.

8

INDUCTION OF OVULATION

1. What is the treatment of anovulation?
It depends on the cause.

In some cases, for example, premature menopause, there is no effective method to induce ovulation and treatment, therefore, is symptomatic with oestrogen replacement therapy.

If the prolactin level is raised, treatment is with bromocriptine unless the cause of the raised prolactin level is thyroid deficiency, in which case replacement therapy with thyroid hormone is given.

If the patient is underweight, the first line of treatment must be to increase body weight. The reason is that pregnancy in underweight women results in the birth of babies that are underweight too. These babies may be immature, born earlier than normal and require forceps deliveries more often than normal, that is, despite being smaller than normal, the babies need help in being delivered. We have found that thin women (BMI below 19 kgs per metre^2, see Chapter 7, question 14) who get pregnant without medical help have twice the rate of underweight babies as do women of normal weight. But we also found that underweight women who had developed amenorrhoea and, therefore, needed treatment to induce ovulation had underweight babies *five* times more often than women of normal weight. Half of the babies born to these mothers were smaller than normal. It is as though developing amenorrhoea is nature's way of stopping women whose metabolism is very vulnerable to subnutrition from getting pregnant.

Since being underweight produces an avoidable risk to the baby's development, we strongly advise against any treatment to induce ovulation until the nutrition of the mother-to-be has improved enough to get her body mass index up to 20 or over. The method of calculating the body mass index and how much weight increase is needed is described in the answer to Chapter 7, question 15.

For most other cases of anovulation, however, the first line of treatment is clomiphene citrate.

2. What is clomiphene and how does it work?

Clomiphene citrate was first used to induce ovulation in 1961 and is still widely used today as the first line of drug treatment for anovulation. Because of its chemical structure, clomiphene acts both as an oestrogen and as an anti-oestrogen, depending on its site of action.

Clomiphene acts on both the hypothalamus and the pituitary gland to induce ovulation. At the hypothalamic level it causes LHRH pulses to be released more frequently, while at the pituitary it makes the cells more sensitive to the action of LHRH (Chapter 1, question 4). The net effect is that the amount of FSH and LH released by the pituitary gland is increased. The increased gonadotrophins then stimulate ovarian follicular development. The tablets are stopped after 5 days and by then the follicle is secreting increasing amounts of oestrogen. When the amount of oestrogen reaches the appropriate level, a mid-cycle surge of LH results and ovulation and the formation of a corpus luteum follow.

Clomiphene may also have a minor direct action on the ovary, making it more sensitive to stimulation by FSH.

3. How is clomiphene taken?

Clomiphene citrate is available in 50 mg tablets.

Usually a course of treatment lasts 5 days and the starting dose is one tablet a day. The day of the cycle on which clomiphene is started is not all that important and some doctors prescribe it from days 2-6, some from days 3-7 and some from days 5–9 of the menstrual cycle. We recommend days 2-6.

If the first course of clomiphene results in ovulation, the same dose is given in the next cycle. If, however, there is no ovulation, the dose is increased to 100 mg a day for 5 days. If ovulation occurs, this dose is continued for subsequent cycles. If, however, ovulation does not occur the patient still carries on with this dose for two or three more cycles. This is because some patients do not ovulate during the first course of clomiphene at 100 mg a day for 5 days but do so in subsequent cycles, despite maintaining the same dose. If the patient does not ovulate after three or four cycles of clomiphene at 100 mg a day for 5 days she is considered to be unresponsive to clomiphene.

An important point — it is important to determine whether *each* cycle of treatment is ovulatory or not, using one or other of the methods described in Chapter 5.

4.   Is it useful to increase the dose of clomiphene above 100 mg a day for 5 days?
No.

There is no scientific evidence to support using a dose of clomiphene of greater than two tablets a day and, in fact, the manufacturers recommend a maximum dose of 100 mg a day for 5 days.

The reason why some people feel that it is useful to give 150, 200 or even 250 mg a day is that sometimes a patient who does not ovulate on 100 mg a day ovulates when given a higher dose. These patients would probably have ovulated if they had been continued on 100 mg for a few more cycles. Increasing the dose of clomiphene does not increase its efficacy but it does lead to more side effects.

5.   What are the side effects of clomiphene?
Clomiphene has few side effects and these occur infrequently.

The most common are thickening of the cervical mucus, making it more difficult for sperm to penetrate, and vaginal dryness. This is one reason why the lowest effective dose of clomiphene should be used. Five percent or so of women who take clomiphene experience hot flushes. Some women develop ovarian cysts. The cysts are not dangerous and disappear once treatment is stopped.

Other symptoms which have been reported occasionally include abdominal bloating, breast discomfort, nausea, skin rash, dizziness and depression.

Very rarely, the patient may experience blurring of vision and, if this occurs, treatment with clomiphene should be stopped.

6.   How successful is clomiphene in inducing ovulation?
Very. Overall, 70-75 percent of women ovulate on clomiphene.

Patients who do not respond well are those with oestrogen deficiency. This group includes patients with hypogonadotrophic hypogonadism, hyperprolactinaemia and premature menopause.

7.   What is the pregnancy rate of patients on clomiphene treatment?
The pregnancy rate of patients on clomiphene therapy is 30-35 percent.

8.   Why is the pregnancy rate of patients on clomiphene therapy so much lower than the ovulation rate?
The exact reason is not known but there are a number of possibilities.

First, the tests of ovulation may have been unreliable and the patients may not actually have ovulated. Second, **ovum entrapment** or a **luteinised unruptured follicle** may have occurred. What this means is that although a corpus luteum has been formed the egg has not been released from the follicle. Third, clomiphene may cause the cervical mucus to become thick so that sperm may be unable to pass through. Fourth, there might be another cause of infertility which has not been treated. Finally, intercourse may have been wrongly timed.

In our experience, the commonest problems are a thick mucus when the dose of clomiphene has been too high and the presence of other, undiagnosed, causes of infertility. These are either tubal problems or persistent hypersecretion of LH in patients with the polycystic ovary syndrome (Chapter 7, question 36). We think that LH should always be measured in patients having clomiphene in at least one cycle of treatment (on about day 8). We also advocate laparoscopy and tubal assessment if the patient has had about six ovulations but still has not conceived.

9.   Does clomiphene cause multiple pregnancy?
Clomiphene causes twin pregnancy in about 5 percent of cases.

The risk rises, therefore, from a natural twining rate of about one in eighty to one in twenty. It very rarely causes triplet or higher order multiple pregnancy.

10.   Does clomiphene increase the risk of miscarriage or abnormal babies?
There is no evidence of an increased risk of abnormal babies.

Miscarriage does seem to occur more frequently in pregnancies conceived as a result of clomiphene therapy. The cause is uncertain but it may be related to the tendency of clomiphene to stimulate LH secretion in patients with polycystic ovary syndrome (Chapter 7, question 36). For this reason we check LH measurements during the 3 or 4 days after the tablets have been stopped and, if the levels are high, change the treatment to tamoxifen (question 12).

11.   What about combining clomiphene and hCG injections?
If clomiphene fails to induce ovulation the reason should be checked by ultrasound scanning of the ovaries. In 80 percent of cases it fails because the follicles do not grow at all, or grow a little but do not reach a pre-ovulatory size. In these cases giving hCG will not produce ovulation.

In 20 percent of cases, however, the follicle grows until it has an average diameter of 17-18 mm but it does not rupture because there is no surge of luteinising hormone. In these cases, an injection of hCG given when the follicle has reached a pre-ovulatory size may trigger ovulation. The timing of hCG injection has to be based on serial ultrasound scans or measurements of the serum oestradiol concentration. If the hCG is given too early the follicle does not rupture but regresses.

12.   What other drugs are there besides clomiphene which induce ovulation?

Besides clomiphene, the other drugs that are sometimes used to induce ovulation are tamoxifen, cyclofenil and epimestrol. They are taken the same way as clomiphene and have a similar sort of action.

13.   If clomiphene fails to induce ovulation, what other treatments are there?

A number of drugs may be used if clomiphene fails to induce ovulation. These are human menopausal gonadotrophin (hMG), follicle stimulating hormone (FSH), pulsatile luteinising hormone releasing hormone (LHRH), and LHRH agonist therapy followed by hMG. In addition, if polycystic ovarian syndrome is responsible for the failure of ovulation, there are surgical procedures such as diathermy of the ovaries (question 50).

14.   What is hMG?

hMG stands for human menopausal gonadotrophin.

It has been used for induction of ovulation since the 1960's. Each ampoule of hMG contains 75 IU of human follicle stimulating hormone (FSH) and an equal amount of human luteinising hormone (LH).

hMG is prepared by extracting gonadotrophins, that is LH and FSH, from the urine of post-menopausal women. It is available in two preparations, called Pergonal and Humegon. They are virtually identical.

15.   How does hMG work?

hMG works by directly stimulating follicles in the ovary.

There is a very fine line between inadequate and excessive stimulation of the ovaries. When it was first introduced, hMG was used to treat all cases of anovulation. It requires intensive monitoring, however, and may cause multiple pregnancy and ovarian hyperstimulation so it is no longer used as first line treatment of anovulation. Nowadays it is reserved for cases in which clomiphene has failed to induce ovulation. The exception is when hMG is deliberately used to stimulate many follicles to develop for IVF or other methods of assisted fertility (see Chapter 11 and 12).

16.   How is hMG given?

hMG is given by intra-muscular injection. The aim in anovulatory women is to stimulate development of a single follicle.

Treatment is started with the lowest dose of hMG that will achieve this. Basically, there are two schedules used. In the first, three equal doses of hMG are given on alternate days with the first injection being given in the first 7 days of the menstrual cycle. In the second regimen, injections of hMG are given every day until an adequate response is obtained. Since most anovulatory women do not ovulate on hMG alone, once an adequate follicular response has been obtained, a single injection of another hormone, human chorionic gonadotrophin (hCG) is given. This mimics the normal mid-cycle surge of LH and causes the follicle to rupture and release the egg. The patient is advised to have sexual intercourse on the day of, and the day after, hCG administration.

In our practice, we always use the second (daily injection) method. We start with one ampoule per day of hMG and, depending on the response, raise the dose every seven to eight days. Once the follicle has started to grow, the same dose is given each day until the hCG is given.

17. How is treatment with hMG monitored?
The problem with hMG is that the dose needed to induce ovulation varies from woman to woman and even from one treatment cycle to the next in the same woman. A slightly inadequate dose of hMG fails to induce ovulation while a slightly excessive dose may cause many follicles to develop, increasing the risk of multiple ovulation, multiple pregnancy and ovarian hyperstimulation.

Careful monitoring of the cycle is, therefore, essential to minimise these risks. Two methods are commonly used, namely, ultrasound scanning of the follicles and measurement of the amount of oestrogen produced by the developing follicle (the measurements can be made on samples of blood or urine). Some infertility specialists use both methods, others use one or the other.

If both methods are used, the first scan and blood test are done on the second day of the menstrual cycle. The ovaries and uterus are scanned, their size and the thickness of the endometrium measured and any cysts in the ovary noted. The second blood test and ultrasound scan are performed on day 8 of treatment. Subsequently, blood tests and ultrasound scans are ideally performed every day until the follicle has an average diameter of 17 mm and the level of oestradiol in the blood is about 1100 pmol/l (300ng/ml). The injection of hCG is given then and an ultrasound scan and measurement of serum progesterone concentration performed 1 week later to make sure a corpus luteum is present.

18. How effective is hMG?
It depends on the type of patient being treated.

If the patient has hypogonadotrophic hypogonadism, hMG is very effective, more than 90 percent of cycles will be ovulatory and the pregnancy rate should be the same as in someone of the same age who ovulates normally.

In the case of polycystic ovarian syndrome, if only patients who have failed to ovulate with clomiphene are considered, 70-75 percent of cycles are ovulatory. The pregnancy rate, however, is much lower, about 30-35 percent.

19. What are the side effects of hMG?

hMG may sometimes cause a little inflammation at the injection site. Rarely, transient fever and joint pains have also been reported.

The two major problems associated with the use of hMG are multiple pregnancy and ovarian hyperstimulation. In most published series the risk of multiple pregnancy is about 25 percent of women who conceive. Although most of these cases are twins, occasionally triplet, quadruplet and even sextuplet pregnancies occur. High order multiple pregnancies have an increased risk of premature labour, miscarriage, high blood pressure, excessive accumulation of amniotic fluid (the fluid that surrounds the baby) and difficult childbirth. Probably the most depressing sequence of events is multiple pregnancy leading to a premature labour, which results in the birth of small and immature babies which have an increased **perinatal mortality** (that is, death of a baby any time between 28 weeks of gestation and 7 days after birth). In the United Kingdom the perinatal mortality of twins is increased threefold and of triplets fivefold.

The other major complication of hMG treatment is ovarian hyperstimulation syndrome (question 20).

The risk of multiple pregnancy and ovarian hyperstimulation syndrome can be greatly reduced when good monitoring is used. For this reason we think hMG treatment should only be undertaken in units with good ultrasound facilities (or access to rapid oestrogen measurements) and experienced personnel. We always withhold the hCG injection in cases where there are more than three follicles with a diameter of 17 mm or more. Using this rule, the multiple pregnancy rate in our unit is 12 percent.

20. What is ovarian hyperstimulation syndrome and what is its treatment?

Ovarian hyperstimulation syndrome is the medical condition that arises when the ovaries have been overstimulated. It usually only occurs after hCG has been given.

There are three degrees of hyperstimulation, namely, mild, moderate and severe. The dangers depend on the grade.

Mild hyperstimulation refers to enlargement of the ovaries, with cyst formation. It occurs in up to 10 percent of cases receiving hMG. As the cysts enlarge, the patient may experience heaviness, abdominal discomfort, swelling and pain. Mild hyperstimulation is not serious. The patient is advised to rest and pain is easily relieved by analgesic drugs such as aspirin.

In moderate hyperstimulation the abdominal discomfort is more severe as the ovarian cysts enlarge. Nausea, vomiting and diarrhoea are present and there is some weight gain. Although patients with moderate hyperstimulation do not require active treatment, they must be closely observed just in case it progresses to severe hyperstimulation.

Severe hyperstimulation is rare (less than 1 percent of cases) but when it does occur, it is serious. Fluid may accumulate in the abdomen and chest, causing difficult breathing and there may be changes in blood clotting which predispose to thrombosis. On very rare occasions it has proved fatal. Treatment involves hospitalisation, with correction of fluid abnormalities.

21. How can the risk of multiple pregnancies and ovarian hyperstimulation be reduced when hMG is used?
The **only way** is by careful monitoring of treatment, using ultrasound scanning of the number and size of the ovarian follicles and/or blood tests to measure the levels of oestrogen.

If there are more than three follicles seen of diameter equal to or greater than 17 mm, or if the oestrogen levels are greater than 2,500 pmol/l, the hCG injection should be withheld and sexual intercourse avoided. Without the hCG injection, the follicles do not normally rupture and the risks of multiple pregnancy and ovarian hyperstimulation are minimised.

22. What is the difference between hMG and purified FSH?
An ampoule of hMG contains equal amounts of FSH and LH, that is, 75 IU each of LH and FSH.

An ampoule of purified FSH, on the other hand, contains 75 IU of FSH but less than 0.4 units of LH.

With regard to their effects, it is debatable whether they produce different results. Our own studies, both in the treatment of anovulatory patients and in ovarian stimulation for IVF, have shown no advantage of using "pure FSH".

23. Can hMG or FSH be given in any other way?
The usual way to give hMG or purified FSH is by daily intra-muscular injections. Some doctors have tried giving them in small intermittent doses by means of a pump. Unlike luteinising hormone releasing hormone (LHRH),

which must be given in a pump for it to work (question 25), with gonadotrophin preparations there is no convincing advantage in pulsatile administration.

24. I have heard that sometimes growth hormone is used for fertility treatment. Can you explain?

For many years little was known about the effects of treatment with growth hormone, other than its ability to make children with certain growth problems grow faster. Now growth hormone is in plentiful supply, we are beginning to learn about its many widespread actions and it appears that it is important in adults as well as in growing children. It seems, for example, that the human ovary can be sensitised to the action of the gonadotrophins by treatment with growth hormone.

In some women with amenorrhoea, the ovarian response to treatment with hMG is poor: large amounts of hMG have to be given, despite which the follicular response is disappointing. Sometimes this occurs in patients with hypogonadotrophic hypogonadism and hypopituitarism. We have found that in these patients the response to treatment with hMG can be improved by additional treatment with growth hormone.

25. What is pulsatile LHRH treatment?

LHRH stands for luteinising hormone releasing hormone; it is a hormone produced in the part of the brain called the hypothalamus (Chapter 1, question 4). It stimulates the pituitary gland to release FSH and LH. LHRH is normally released from the hypothalamus in minute quantities at regular intervals, one pulse every 60-90 minutes. It is not released continuously.

Pulsatile LHRH treatment is a method of inducing ovulation in which small quantities of LHRH are given to the patient at regular intervals to mimic the normal pattern of release from the hypothalamus. It is used for patients who do not ovulate even in response to treatment with clomiphene citrate and, ideally, who have hypogonadotrophic hypogonadism. It is not the correct treatment for hyperprolactinaemia and does not work in patients with a premature menopause.

26. Why must LHRH be given in a pump?

Because for LHRH to work it has to be given in a way that mimics its normal secretion. It cannot be taken by mouth because it would be digested by the acid in the stomach and it is obviously impractical to administer an injection every hour and a half.

These small battery powered pumps can be set to inject the LHRH every one and a half hours. The LHRH is dissolved in a solution which is contained in

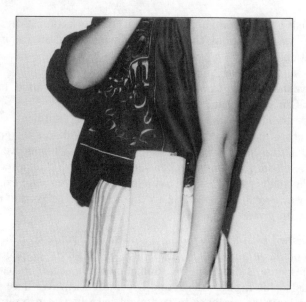

Figure 8.1 This shows a patient wearing an LHRH pump. The pump is concealed underneath the clothes and the very fine needle is inserted subcutaneously in the upper arm.

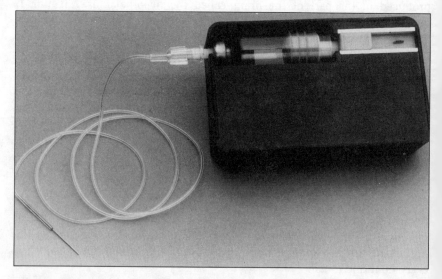

Figure 8.2 A close-up view of the LHRH pump with the infusion set. The pump delivers small doses of LHRH at regular intervals and is used in the treatment of anovulatory infertility.

a syringe that is placed inside the pump. The patient wears the pump on a belt around the waist (Figure 8.1). The belt can easily be concealed beneath clothes. The syringe is connected to an infusion set, which runs underneath the clothes. It has a tiny needle which is inserted subcutaneously just beneath the skin of the outer part of the upper arm (Figure 8.2). Every 1.5 hours, the pump injects a few drops of LHRH into the body.

Note that the needle is placed subcutaneously; one gets used to it very quickly — after all, patients with diabetes have to inject themselves subcutaneously two or three times a day.

Some doctors place the needle directly into a vein. This brings with it certain problems (the LHRH solution has to contain some anticoagulant to prevent the needle from becoming blocked by clotted blood, the needle cannot be adjusted by the patient herself and the risk of infection has always to be considered). We hardly ever administer the LHRH intravenously, finding the subcutaneous route satisfactory for nine out of ten patients.

27. Do I have to wear the pump all the time?
More or less all the time, because LHRH is normally released day and night. There are, of course, intervals of an hour and a half when the pump is not working, so the pump can be removed then. It is, for example, essential to take it off when bathing or showering because it is easily damaged by water.

Most patients remove and replace the pump themselves. Although it seems inconvenient at the beginning, you will find that you learn to adjust very quickly to its use.

28. How many different types of pump are there?
There are many different brands (Figure 8.3) but they all act in more or less the same way. The size varies but is usually just larger than a packet of kingsize cigarettes.

29. Does the pump take over control of my body?
No, all the pump does is to administer the LHRH intermittently. It has no other effect on the body.

30. Do I have to be admitted into hospital for treatment?
No, the treatment is entirely on an outpatient basis.

31. How is LHRH pump therapy monitored?
Before treatment is started, the patient is given a full explanation of how the pump works. A contact telephone number is given in case of a mechanical problem over a weekend (for example, the pump battery running out).

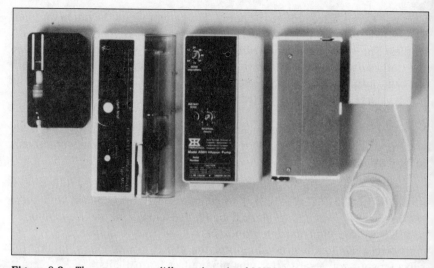

Figure 8.3 There are many different brands of LHRH pumps available as shown in this photograph.

Most people find using the pump very simple and are able to change syringes and needles themselves. We have treated more than 200 patients in over 600 cycles of treatment and none of our patients has ever had to give up therapy because of practical difficulties with the pump. When the needle is properly placed, one should feel no pain or discomfort throughout the full range of arm movements.

Once the pump has been fitted, monitoring of treatment is by ultrasound alone. There is no need for blood tests except for research purposes. After an ultrasound scan on the day the pump is fitted, the second scan is scheduled on day 10 of treatment and then on alternate days until ovulation occurs. Providing the response to treatment in the first cycle is ovulatory, monitoring in subsequent cycles can be restricted to a single measurement of serum progesterone on day 21.

32. How often do the syringes and needles have to be changed?
Each syringe of LHRH lasts for about 4 days or so. The entire infusion set is changed whenever a new syringe of LHRH is used.

33. What happens if the pump fails?
All the pumps used for LHRH treatment are made with excellent mechanical and electronic components and pump failure is unusual. The most common reason for pump failure is a flat battery. Most pumps have a low battery

warning device which allows plenty of notice before the pump stops. You should keep a spare battery and know how to connect it.

In the unlikely event that the pump fails for some other reason, you should contact your treatment centre for further advice as soon as possible. Provided the pump is changed for another one quickly, the treatment is generally not affected. Pump failure is not dangerous — the worst that can happen is that a cycle of treatment has to be abandoned.

34. Can I continue working while I am on treatment?
Yes, you can.

Wearing the pump does not interfere with your lifestyle in any way. You can continue working and take part in sports. The only exception is swimming. If you do go swimming, you should remove the pump after it has administered a dose of LHRH and put it on again before one and a half hours have elapsed.

35. What is the success rate of LHRH pump treatment?
It depends on the type of patient treated.

In cases of hypogonadotrophic hypogonadism, the success rate is excellent, more than 90 percent of cycles are ovulatory and after 6 months 90 percent of the women are pregnant.

In the case of polycystic ovary syndrome, the ovulatory rate in patients who have not ovulated on treatment with clomiphene is about 50 percent and the cumulative conception rate (Chapter 4, question 15) is about 50 percent at 6 months. The ovulatory rate in polycystic ovary syndrome can be raised if clomiphene or a small dose of FSH is given as well (question 43). One feature worth noting when LHRH is used for polycystic ovary syndrome is that treatment is much less effective if the woman is over-weight. Moreover, it sometimes takes more than 20 days of treatment before there is satisfactory follicular development. It is, therefore, important to give pulsatile LHRH for up to 4 weeks before a failure to respond is diagnosed. Lastly, there is evidence that subcutaneous LHRH is more effective when it is injected into the upper arm than when it is given into the abdominal wall.

36. What side effects are there with pump therapy?
Virtually none when it is used subcutaneously. Occasionally, a mild local infection occurs at the needle site. This is easily treated by re-siting the needle; occasionally a course of antibiotics is required.

If LHRH is given intravenously, there is a very small risk of septicaemia, that is, of an infection in the blood stream. This risk is probably more theoretical than real but we prefer to reduce it even further by restricting the intravenous route to those who definitely do not respond to subcutaneous therapy and who do not want to use hMG.

37. How much does LHRH pump treatment cost and how does the price compare with hMG treatment?

The cost of LHRH pump treatment is the sum of the price of the pump, the cost of the hormone itself and the cost of monitoring. Although the initial cost of the pump may be expensive, it can of course be used by many patients. We have had some pumps in almost continual use for 4 years. The cost of monitoring is much less than when hMG is used.

One study compared directly how much it costs with the two forms of treatment — pulsatile LHRH worked out to be cheaper.

38. What are the advantages of LHRH pump treatment compared with hMG treatment?

The major advantage is safety.

The risk of ovarian hyperstimulation is almost non-existent compared with the 1 percent rate of severe and 10 percent rate of mild hyperstimulation associated with hMG treatment.

Although wearing a pump is inconvenient, most people get used to it very quickly and there is the compensation of not needing the large number of blood tests and ultrasound scans that are obligatory with hMG treatment.

39. Is there any risk of multiple pregnancy?

The risk of multiple pregnancy is very much lower than with hMG treatment — 3-6 percent for twins (depending on whether hCG is given at mid-cycle) and 1 percent for triplets; higher order multiple pregnancies are virtually unheard of with LHRH treatment.

40. Is there any risk of ovarian hyperstimulation?

No.

41. Is there any increased risk of abnormal babies?

No.

42. If I have a baby with LHRH treatment, does it mean I will need LHRH to become pregnant again?

Not necessarily so.

Some patients resume spontaneous ovulation after childbirth while others regain the response to clomiphene. If, however, you have hypogonadotrophic hypogonadism, you will almost certainly need to have pulsatile LHRH therapy again to get pregnant.

43.   If subcutaneous pulsatile LHRH fails to induce ovulation, is there anything that can be done to improve its success?
There are two techniques that can be used - the first is to combine treatment with pulsatile LHRH and treatment with clomiphene (at a dose of 100 mg a day for 5 days). This improves the response in perhaps half of the cases of polycystic ovary syndrome that have not responded to either form of treatment alone. The mechanism of the interaction is uncertain but it may represent the action of clomiphene increasing the responsiveness of the pituitary to the injected LHRH.

If combined pulsatile LHRH and clomiphene does not work, a small dose of purified FSH can be given intra-muscularly for a few days to augment the effect on the ovary of the gonadotrophins secreted in response to the treatment with pulsatile LHRH. This combination will improve the response in just over half of the patients with polycystic ovary syndrome who have not re-sponded to all of the above treatments.

44.   What is the advantage of augmenting the effect of pulsatile LHRH in this way as compared with just using hMG or FSH alone?
The main advantage of such a stepwise approach is that the risk of multiple pregnancy and ovarian hyperstimulation is minimised.

45.   What are LHRH analogues and what is the difference between them and pulsatile LHRH?
So far we have been describing the use of natural LHRH, that is, LHRH which is identical to the LHRH that the brain normally produces. Natural LHRH has to be given in a pulsatile fashion for it to work. It is, however, possible to alter the chemical structure of natural LHRH so that the new molecule has some of the activities of the parent molecule but some new ones too.

Such compounds are called LHRH analogues. They may differ from natural LHRH by as little as one aminoacid (there are ten aminoacids (building blocks) in the naturally occurring LHRH molecule). A variety of compounds have been made and include buserelin, nafarelin, decapeptyl and zoladex.

When LHRH analogues are given they start by stimulating the pituitary gland but after a few days of continuous use they desensitise the pituitary, that is, it no longer responds to the analogue or the natural LHRH from the hypothalamus. The output of FSH and LH thereby falls. LHRH analogues therefore inhibit the patient's pituitary from producing its own FSH and LH so the ovary becomes quiescent. It can then be stimulated by giving the pa-tient injections of hMG or purified FSH.

The reason for using this approach is that failure of ovulation and conception may be associated with excessive secretion of LH by the patient's own pituitary (Chapter 7, question 34). By suppressing its over-secretion and then giving injections of hMG or FSH one hopes to eliminate this problem. This approach can also be used in ovarian stimulation for IVF (Chapter 11, question 5).

46. How is LHRH analogue and hMG treatment given?

Treatment with the LHRH analogue is started either in the middle of the luteal phase or at the beginning of the menstrual cycle. The most commonly used analogue is buserelin. Unfortunately it cannot be given by mouth because it gets digested by the acid in the stomach so it is given either as a nasal spray (sniffed four to six times a day) or by daily subcutaneous injections.

After 2 weeks of treatment an ultrasound scan is performed and the oestradiol level is measured. If it is low, and the ultrasound scan shows that the follicles are small and the uterine endometrium thin, it indicates that pituitary secretion of LH and FSH has been adequately suppressed. Treatment with daily injections of hMG is then started while the buserelin is continued. When the largest follicle has grown sufficiently to ovulate (that is, to a diameter of 16-20 mm), an injection of hCG is given to rupture the follicle. Treatment with buserelin is stopped after the hCG injection.

47. Is LHRH analogue and hMG treatment more successful than hMG alone?

At the present time the evidence suggests that LHRH analogue and hMG treatment is no more effective than hMG alone in inducing ovulation. The risk of ovarian hyperstimulation and multiple pregnancy is also not reduced. The only question unresolved is whether the miscarriage rate is lowered by the use of LHRH analogue because the patient's own production of LH is suppressed (Chapter 7, question 36).

48. What are the surgical treatments that may be used to induce ovulation in polycystic ovarian disease?

The two operations are wedge resection of the ovaries and diathermy of the ovaries.

49. Is wedge resection of the ovaries a good operation?

Wedge resection of the ovaries involves an abdominal operation in which a wedge of ovarian tissue is removed from both ovaries. The cut edges are then sewn back together.

This operation was the first treatment to be used in patients with polycystic ovary syndrome. It is effective in restoring ovulation in about 70 percent of cases. The trouble is that, if the ovaries bleed, scarring and adhesions may form around the fallopian tubes so that they become blocked. Since clomiphene became available for induction of ovulation, there has been little place for this operation.

50.   Can you tell me something about electrodiathermy and laser treatment to induce ovulation in polycystic ovary syndrome?
When it was realised that the cause of the adhesions was bleeding some surgeons proposed that the operation be done using electro-diathermy — this is the instrument used by surgeons to stop bleeding from small blood vessels. It has been found that, using electrodiathermy or the laser, four small burns to each of the ovaries has about the same effect as surgical removal of a wedge of ovary.

The advantage of this procedure is that it is done through the laparoscope. This means the patient is only in the hospital for one night. Like wedge resection it increases the rate of ovulation and lowers serum LH levels. We do not yet know the mechanism by which it works.

In our practice, we reserve ovarian diathermy for slim patients (being overweight makes the operation technically more difficult) who have a persistently elevated serum LH concentration and who have not responded to treatment with clomiphene or tamoxifen.

9

ENDOMETRIOSIS

1. What is endometriosis?

Endometriosis is a condition seen in women of reproductive age in which endometrial tissue, which is the normal lining of the uterus, is found outside the uterus. The areas commonly affected are the ovaries, fallopian tubes, surface of the uterus and the walls of the pelvis.

The condition is mostly seen in women between 30 and 40 years of age. It is related to delayed childbearing, in the sense that women who have children when they are relatively young seldom get endometriosis. Endometriosis is commonly associated with painful menstrual periods, painful intercourse and infertility.

2. How common is endometriosis?

It is responsible for 20 percent or so of cases of infertility.

3. What causes endometriosis?

The cause is not fully known.

At the time of normal menstruation, some menstrual blood and cells escape from the uterus through the fallopian tubes into the abdominal cavity. For reasons that we do not understand, in women who get endometriosis, these cells implant in areas outside the uterus. Since these cells come from the endometrial tissue, they respond to the hormonal changes during the menstrual cycle and bleed at the time of menstruation, just like the normal lining of the uterus. Unlike the normal menstrual contents, however, which can flow freely out of the uterus, blood released by the endometriotic tissue has no place to go and is, therefore, reabsorbed into the blood stream. In the process, it leads to inflammation and then scarring. If the scarring is extensive, adhesions form which bind the structures in the pelvis together, distorting their normal anatomical relationship.

4. How does endometriosis cause infertility?

Endometriosis is usually classified as minimal, mild, moderate or severe.

In severe endometriosis, the fallopian tubes, ovaries and bowel are stuck together almost as if a pot of glue had been poured into the pelvis. Release of the egg from the ovary and its passage through the distorted fallopian tube is, therefore, hampered. In the case of milder endometriosis, the manner by which endometriosis is related to infertility is not so clear, although there does appear to be a definite correlation between the two conditions.

5. What symptoms does endometriosis produce?

Endometriosis varies in severity and in about a third of cases the only symptom is infertility. Some women suffer from painful periods (dysmenorrhoea) while others experience painful sexual intercourse (dyspareunia) or abnormal menstrual bleeding. In the case of dysmenorrhoea, the pain often lasts throughout the period of menstrual flow and may even get more painful as menstruation progresses. This is different from the pain that occurs as a result of normal ovulation, when the pain normally disappears after the first day of menstruation.

One important thing to remember, though, is that the severity of symptoms and the extent of endometriosis are not closely correlated so that patients with mild endometriosis may suffer very painful periods while others who have more severe endometriosis may have no symptoms at all.

6. How is endometriosis diagnosed?

By the combination of symptoms, physical examination (the ligaments at the back of the uterus may feel nodular or tender) and laparoscopy. Laparoscopy is the most important diagnostic test since the clinical picture of endometriosis can often be confused with other conditions.

7. What are the different stages of endometriosis?

Classification of the stage of endometriosis is made at the time of laparoscopy. There are a number of different classification systems but the most widely used nowadays is the revised American Fertility Society classification. In this system endometriosis is classified as minimal, mild, moderate or severe (Figure 9.1).

8. What is the treatment of endometriosis?

The most effective treatment is to stop menstruation completely, as occurs naturally during pregnancy or after the menopause. In practice, there are five ways to manage endometriosis, namely, no treatment except for painkilling (analgesic) drugs, hormonal treatment, surgery, a combination of hormonal treatment and surgery and, finally, in-vitro fertilisation (test-tube baby) treat-

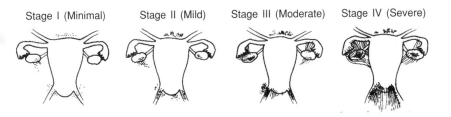

Figure 9.1 Endometriosis is classifield into 4 stages according to its severity.

ment. The last form of treatment does not itself cure the disease but overcomes the problem of infertility.

9. What types of surgery are carried out for endometriosis?

The type of surgery performed depends on the extent of the endometriosis and the symptoms the patient suffers. If the patient has completed her family and the endometriosis is severe and causes very distressing symptoms, major surgery may be necessary to remove both the uterus and ovaries. Once hormone secretion from the ovaries ceases, endometriosis resolves spontaneously.

In the case of infertile patients, if the endometriosis is severe and the adhesions and scarring extensive, the endometriotic implants can either be removed or cauterised, while the adhesions are freed to restore the normal anatomical relationship of the pelvic organs. Such operations can either be performed through an open abdominal operation called a laparotomy or as a laparoscopic procedure. The overall success of infertility surgery for endometriosis is about 60 percent. The main advantage of surgery compared with drug treatment is that the patient can try for a baby within a few weeks of the operation.

10 Can you tell me something about the use of lasers for treating endometriosis?

Laser surgery is a relatively new method of surgery where a laser beam is directed through a laparoscopic probe to burn away the endometriotic implants and divide the adhesions. The major advantage of laser surgery is that it is very precise and the risk of subsequent adhesion formation is lower than with conventional surgery. Laser surgery, however, requires special training and the equipment is very expensive so that it can only be obtained in highly specialised centres.

11. What are the hormonal drugs that can be used to treat endometriosis?

Although a variety of hormonal drugs, including the birth control pill and progesterone-like drugs such as norethisterone, have been used to treat endometriosis, the two most widely used are danazol and analogues of luteinising hormone releasing hormone (LHRH analogues) such as buserelin, zoladex and nafarelin (see question 15).

12.　How does danazol work?

Danazol is a synthetic by-product of the male hormone, testosterone. It suppresses the pituitary gland and ovaries so that a temporary "menopause" is induced. The drug may also have a direct action on endometriotic tissue.

During the artificial menopausal state, the endometriosis regresses and, in most cases, when the drug is stopped 6 months later and menstruation resumes, the endometriosis remains suppressed. It may, however, recur in 30-40 percent of cases within the next 1-4 years of follow up.

13. How effective is danazol?

Its efficacy depends on the stage of the endometriosis. Approximately 30 percent of women with severe endometriosis and 60 percent with mild endometriosis will conceive after danazol treatment.

14.　What are the side effects of danazol and what are the disadvantages of using it?

There are two major problems with danazol treatment.

The first is that danazol suppresses ovulation and the patient, therefore, cannot get pregnant for the 6 months during which the drug is being used. This is a major problem, especially for older women who may have only a short time left to conceive.

The second is that there is a relatively high incidence of side effects. Roughly 20 percent of women on danazol therapy experience side effects. Those that have been reported include weight gain, nausea, blood stained vaginal discharge, hair loss, acne, hot flushes, loss of breast tissue and dryness of the vagina during sexual intercourse. The symptoms are reversible once the drug is stopped, except for hoarseness of voice which is a rare complication but one which does persist once it occurs.

15.　How do LHRH analogues work?

LHRH analogues are drugs in which there is a slight modification of the structure of the LHRH hormone so that their administration suppresses pituitary secretion of LH and FSH. The fall in gonadotrophin secretion affects the ovary, causing menstrual cycles to stop completely. Like danazol, the drugs have to be used continuously for 6 months to be effective. Once the drugs are stopped, menstruation resumes.

Overall, approximately 50 percent of infertile patients with endometriosis become pregnant after treatment with an LHRH analogue. The recurrence rate seems to be similar to that observed after treatment with danazol.

16. How do you use LHRH analogues?

There are a number of different LHRH analogues and they are used differently. Some are given as daily injections or by sniffing for example, buserelin, while others are given as depot injections once a month (zoladex).

17. What side effects do LHRH analogues produce?

The efficacy of LHRH analogues is about the same as for danazol but their major advantage is that they produce fewer side effects.

The main side effects are those caused by oestrogen deficiency, such as hot flushes and dryness of the vagina during intercourse. There may be some decalcification of the bones (osteoporosis) and, on average, there is about a 5 percent loss of bone calcium over 6 months. In most patients, this loss of calcium reverses spontaneously once the LHRH analogue treatment is stopped and the bones return to their pretreatment state.

These problems can be prevented by using small doses of the analogues and by adding treatment with a small dose of a progestogen, such as norethisterone acetate, to the LHRH analogue therapy. We advise this treatment particularly in women with other risk factors for osteoporosis who require treatment with an LHRH analogue. This is something you should discuss with your doctor.

18. Does stopping my menstrual periods harm my body?

No, it does not. It should not be imagined that the treatment stops menstruation by causing a pool of menstrual blood to be stored in the body waiting to be released!

What actually happens is that the pituitary and ovarian hormones are suppressed so that the lining of the uterus does not thicken and there is, therefore, nothing formed which needs to be shed.

19. Can endometriosis recur after treatment?

Endometriosis may recur after treatment in 30-40 percent of cases and some of these patients may require surgical removal of the uterus (hysterectomy) and ovaries.

10

BLOCKED TUBES

1. What causes tubal damage?
By far the commonest cause is infection.

This infection, called pelvic inflammatory disease, may be caused by a variety of bacteria, most of which are common germs we all carry in our bodies. The reasons why these bacteria should cause pelvic inflammatory disease and tubal damage in some women are not completely understood but there are a number of predisposing factors. Women who have had multiple sexual partners, who have used an intra-uterine contraceptive device (IUCD or coil), who have had an infection after a termination of pregnancy or those who have had a ruptured appendix in the past have a higher risk of damaged tubes than normal.

A few women are born with abnormal development or even blockage of one or both tubes while others have tubal damage as a result of scarring and adhesions caused by previous pelvic surgery or endometriosis.

Many women suffering from infertility undergo operations to suspend their uterus (ventro-suspension), remove small fibroids (myomectomy) or have a piece of their ovary removed (wedge resection). The indications for many of these operations are questionable and these operations may themselves sometimes impair subsequent fertility by causing adhesions or distorting the tubes.

2. How does tubal damage cause infertility?
Two ways.

First, the tubes may become blocked so that the eggs are unable to pass through. Second, there may be adhesions which distort the shape of the tubes and their relationship with the ovaries. When this happens egg pick-up by the tubes and the movement of the egg down the tube may be impaired.

3. What percentage of infertile women have damaged tubes?
The figures vary from one country to another and range from 10 percent to
50 percent or more. In most Western countries, surveys suggest that roughly
30 percent of infertile women have tubal problems.

**4. How does pelvic inflammatory disease manifest itself? Does it always
lead to damaged tubes?**
Pelvic inflammatory disease may occur as an acute or a chronic infection.

When it occurs as an acute infection, the patient usually has a fever, pelvic
pain, unpleasant smelling vaginal discharge and heavy periods. Most cases of
pelvic infection that lead to damaged tubes start, however, as chronic infections which slowly damage the tubes and the patient may not even be aware
that it has occurred. The correct treatment for pelvic inflammatory disease is
early, adequate and appropriate antibiotic therapy.

5. How would I know if I have tubal damage?
The groups of patients at high risk have been mentioned above. However, even
if a patient has a history of pelvic inflammatory disease, it does not mean that
she definitely has damaged tubes. On the other hand, as mentioned, many
patients who have damaged tubes have no symptoms or signs at all. Therefore,
all patients who have had difficulty conceiving should have their tubes
checked at some stage of their infertility work-up.

The two tests most often used to diagnose tubal problems are the
hysterosalpingogram (Chapter 5, question 33) and laparoscopy (Chapter 5,
question 37).

6. What types of operations are there to correct damaged tubes?
The type of operation depends on the nature of the tubal damage. The commonest problem is the presence of adhesions around the tubes. In such cases,
an operation called **adhesiolysis** or **salpingolysis** can be performed to divide
the adhesions. There are different ways of performing adhesiolysis, either at
the time of laparoscopy using a tiny pair of scissors or by laser surgery, or
through a separate operation. The success rate of adhesiolysis varies from 35-
60 percent, depending on the severity of the adhesions.

If a portion of the tube is blocked but both ends are healthy, the blocked
portion can be removed and the healthy portions joined together. The pregnancy rate following such operations varies according to the extent of tubal
blockage, the site of blockage and the type of surgery used. For example, when
microsurgical techniques are used for reversal of a previous sterilisation operation the pregnancy rate is as high as 55-75 percent.

On the other hand, if the blockage occurs near the cornual end of the tube (that is, next to its entrance to the uterus) and a tubo-cornual anastomosis performed, the pregnancy rate is only about 30-55 percent.

Sometimes, there is total blockage of the outer end of the tube but the rest of the tube is patent (this is called a **hydrosalpinx).** In such cases an operation **(salpingostomy)** may be performed to open up the tube (Figure 10.1). This leads to a pregnancy in about 18-30 percent of cases. Finally, if the blockage occurs where the tube joins the uterus and the damage extends right through

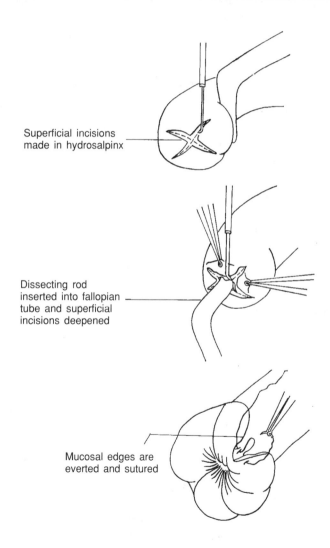

Superficial incisions made in hydrosalpinx

Dissecting rod inserted into fallopian tube and superficial incisions deepened

Mucosal edges are everted and sutured

Figure 10.1 Salpingostomy.

the wall of the uterus, a new hole can be bored into the uterus and the tube reimplanted through this opening. This operation is called **tubal implantation** and carries a 25 percent chance of success.

7.   What is microsurgery?
Microsurgery refers to the use of an operating microscope to help in the infertility surgery. The microscope is invaluable because the fallopian tube is very tiny and, at its narrowest part, its internal diameter is only 0.5 mm. Using a microscope, the surgeon can stitch the tube more accurately while avoiding damage to the surrounding delicate tissues, thus reducing the risk of adhesion formation after the surgery.

8.   What factors affect the success rate of operations for tubal damage?
The success rates depend on the extent and site of tubal damage, the age of the patient, the presence or absence of any other causes of infertility, the skill of the surgeon and the type of operation performed. In general, microsurgery and laser surgery offer the best chances of success and the pregnancy rates following the different operations have been given above.

9.   Can my tubes get blocked again after tubal surgery?
This is possible in a minority of cases.

With microsurgery, the risk is about 10 percent compared with about 40 percent when conventional surgery is used. One thing that you should note, though, is that even if the tube remains open it does not always mean that pregnancy can be achieved. Sometimes, the lining of the tubes have been damaged so badly that they can no longer work effectively even though they are completely open.

10.   Can I get pregnant if I only have one healthy tube?
Yes, although you are likely to get pregnant more quickly if both tubes are healthy.

11.   If my tubes are blocked, can I have them replaced with artificial tubes?
As described previously, the fallopian tube is a complex structure and is not simply a pipe through which the egg travels into the uterus. The tube helps to pick up the egg after ovulation, transports both sperm and eggs and allows an optimum environment for fertilisation to occur and early development of the embryo to take place. It cannot be replaced by artificial tubes.

12.   If I have been sterilised, can I still have a child?
It depends on the way the sterilisation was performed. If it was performed by electrodiathermy, that is, burning of the tubes, and the damage is very exten-

sive, the chance of successful tubal surgery is very small and it is much better to have test-tube baby treatment instead. On the other hand, if the sterilisation was by means of a clip which seals off the middle part of the tube, reversal of sterilisation by microsurgery is very successful and the majority of patients (55-75 percent) will achieve pregnancy.

13. Will I be able to give birth normally after tubal surgery?
In most cases, you can. The only exception is if you have had a tubal implantation. In such cases, the wall of the uterus may be weakened and it is often advisable to have a Caesarean section.

14. Is there a higher risk of ectopic pregnancy after reversal of sterilisation?
Yes. There is a higher risk of ectopic pregnancy (pregnancy implanting outside the uterus) after all types of tubal surgery. This is mainly because when the tubes are damaged, their lining is often damaged as well and although the tubes may be opened up by surgery, the fertilised egg does not pass through them as easily as if the tubes were healthy. There is, therefore, a higher chance that the embryo may implant in the tube instead of passing down into the uterus.

11

TEST TUBE BABIES, EMBRYO FREEZING AND EGG DONATION

1. What is IVF?

IVF stands for in-vitro fertilisation, commonly known as test-tube baby treatment.

The basic principle involves removing one or more mature eggs (the medical term for eggs is oocytes) from the ovary, fertilising them outside the body, using sperm either from the partner or from a donor and then transferring one or more of the fertilised eggs back into the uterus.

The procedure whereby embryos are transferred into the uterus is called embryo transfer, often referred to as ET.

Recently, the preferred medical term for a fertilised egg has become "pre-embryo"; after 2 weeks the term used is "embryo". This terminology fits in with the stages of development, because the streak of tissue which ultimately develops into the nervous system can first be identified 14 days after fertilisation.

2. Who needs IVF?

When IVF was invented by Mr Patrick Steptoe and Dr (now Professor) Robert Edwards in 1978, it was first used to help women with blocked fallopian tubes because in these cases the sperm and egg cannot meet naturally. Even today, more than half of the patients who have IVF do so because they have blocked tubes or because their tubes are so badly damaged that tubal surgery cannot help. It has also been found, however, that IVF can be used to help couples who have infertility problems caused by endometriosis, low sperm counts or sperm defects, male and female antibody problems or even when the infertility is "unexplained".

While just over 7,500 women underwent treatment by IVF in the United Kingdom in 1988, according to one study approximately 20 percent of all infertile couples will benefit from treatment by IVF.

3. What are the steps involved in IVF?
There are five basic steps:

a) Stimulation of the ovaries so that several follicles are produced.

b) Monitoring the growth of the follicles and deciding when the eggs are mature enough for collection. At this stage, an injection of a hormone called hCG (human chorionic gonadotrophin) is given to cause final maturation of the eggs.

c) The egg collection procedure. Eggs are usually collected using ultrasound techniques although some centres practise egg collection by laparoscopy. Egg collection is timed for 34-36 hours after the hCG injection.

d) Fertilisation of the eggs in the laboratory.

e) Transferring one or more pre-embryos back into the uterus.

4. What is the advantage of stimulating the ovaries to produce many eggs?
When IVF was first used successfully, a single egg was obtained during a natural menstrual cycle and drugs were not given to stimulate follicular development. It was later found that the pregnancy rate was higher when several rather than just one pre-embryo was transferred. Since then, it has become standard practice in most IVF programmes to give the patient drugs to stimulate the ovaries so that several follicles develop. In this way, it is hoped that several eggs will be collected so that several pre-embryos will be available for transfer.

In the last few years, this has become even more important because it is now possible to freeze pre-embryos. These "spare" pre-embryos can then be transferred into the uterus in a subsequent cycle and the patient does not have to go through the ovarian stimulation and egg collection procedures again.

5. How are the ovaries stimulated to produce several eggs?
Two methods are commonly used.

The first is to stimulate the ovaries with human menopausal gonadotrophin (hMG) with or without clomiphene citrate. If both are given together, then a typical protocol is for the patient to take two tablets of clomiphene daily from the second to the sixth day of the menstrual cycle. hMG injections are given every day starting from the fourth day of the menstrual cycle.

The second method is to use an LHRH analogue together with hMG. The purpose of using an LHRH analogue is to stop the patient from producing

FSH and LH herself so that stimulation of the ovaries is completely controlled. The LHRH analogue treatment also prevents a pre-ovulatory LH surge from occurring so that spontaneous ovulation (before egg collection) is avoided.

There are two protocols available for giving LHRH analogues. In the "long" protocol, the LHRH analogue is given for 7-14 days to desensitise the patient's pituitary gland and prevent it from releasing FSH and LH. Once desensitisation has occurred, which occasionally takes more than 2 weeks, daily injections of hMG are added to stimulate the ovaries. Both LHRH analogue and hMG are then continued until the eggs are mature enough for egg collection to be undertaken.

In the "short" protocol of LHRH analogue administration, treatment with both the LHRH analogue and the hMG is started at the beginning of the menstrual cycle.

6.   Do these drugs produce any side effects?
The drugs are very safe and generally produce no major side effects unless too high a dose is used.

In about 1 percent of cases, excessive stimulation of the ovaries occurs and ovarian hyperstimulation severe enough to require hospitalisation results. With regard to minor side effects, the ones commonly experienced are hot flushes and vaginal dryness because of the LHRH analogue. These side affects are transient.

7.   What is the ovarian hyperstimulation syndrome in IVF?
It is basically the same as the ovarian hyperstimulation that can complicate normal induction of ovulation (Chapter 8, question 20).

In IVF the condition is far less common than one would expect, considering the relatively large amounts of drugs given to stimulate the ovaries. The reason is thought to be that during egg collection the follicles are emptied of their follicular fluid as well as their eggs.

Nevertheless the syndrome can occur in IVF and the symptoms are the same as in induction of ovulation. In mild cases, the woman has a feeling of abdominal heaviness, swelling and pain. In moderate hyperstimulation, abdominal discomfort is more pronounced and nausea and vomiting and occasionally diarrhoea occur. In severe cases, fluid may collect in the abdominal and chest cavities and there may be difficulty in breathing. There may also be problems with blood clotting and the kidneys failing to produce urine. Fortunately, however, such cases are very rare.

Mild and moderate hyperstimulation do not require any active therapy other than observation and symptomatic treatment. Patients with severe hyperstimulation need hospitalisation and prompt treatment.

8.   What are the main advantages and disadvantages of using LHRH analogues and hMG compared with clomiphene and hMG for ovarian stimulation?

The main advantage of using an LHRH analogue is that it prevents spontaneous ovulation. Consequently, the timing of hCG administration is not so crucial and it is usually possible to schedule egg collection for a time that is convenient for both the patient and the IVF team (for example, avoiding an egg collection at the weekend).

Another advantage is that if there are only one or two large follicles but several smaller ones trailing behind, one can wait a few more days for the smaller follicles to increase in size. There are other possible advantages of using LHRH analogues, such as for patients who have polycystic ovary syndrome (particularly those with high LH concentrations (Chapter 7, question 36)) or who have not responded well to stimulation with clomiphene and hMG. These other advantages have not been proven, however, and a lot of research regarding this is still going on.

The main disadvantage of using hMG with an LHRH analogue rather than with clomiphene is that the duration of treatment is lengthened and the amount of hMG needed to stimulate the ovaries increased. The cost of treatment is therefore increased.

9.   How is the growth of the follicles monitored?

In two ways — by ultrasound scanning of the ovaries and by blood or urine tests to measure the amount of oestrogen produced.

In general, daily ultrasound scans and blood tests are done, starting from about day 6-8 of the cycle. When LHRH analogues are given, however, some centres try to reduce the amount of monitoring. At each ultrasound scan, the number and size of the follicles are measured.

In clomiphene and hMG cycles, when the largest follicle has an average diameter of 17 mm with at least two other follicles of more than 14 mm diameter and a satisfactory oestrogen level, we give an injection of hCG to achieve final maturation of the eggs (Figure 11.1). Timing of the hCG injection is not so critical when LHRH analogues are used.

Eggs are collected 34-36 hours after the injection of hCG.

10.   What happens if I ovulate before the eggs are collected?

In a small proportion of cases (less than 10 percent), when hMG and clomiphene are used to stimulate the ovaries, ovulation occurs before the egg

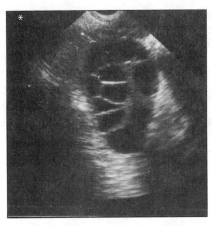

Figure 11.1 This shows an enlarged ovary with multiple ovarian follicles. It is typically seen in patients undergoing test-tube baby (IVF) treatment.

collection is performed. If this happens, the collection is not carried out and the cycle of treatment is usually abandoned. If, however, the patient has patent fallopian tubes and there were four or fewer large follicles seen on the ultrasound scan on the day of hCG administration, it may be possible to change to another procedure called DIPI (Chapter 12, question 13) or to perform intrauterine insemination (Chapter 14, question 15).

If spontaneous ovulation occurs in an IVF treatment cycle, in the next treatment cycle it is a good idea to use the combination of an LHRH analogue and hMG to stimulate the ovaries.

11. What happens if I do not produce several follicles?
If there are fewer than three mature follicles seen on the ultrasound scan, treatment is usually abandoned and, in the next cycle, a different stimulation regimen used or a larger dose of hMG given. In a few cases, however, if it is believed that the patient is unlikely to produce a larger number of follicles even if she were to try another cycle, the doctor may still agree to go ahead with the egg collection, provided that is what the patient wants.

12. How are the eggs collected?
There are two ways: through laparoscopy or by an ultrasound guided procedure.

13. How is laparoscopic egg collection performed?
The technique of laparoscopy has been described (Chapter 5, question 37). The procedure is usually performed as a day case, meaning that the patient is admitted to hospital but is not required to stay overnight.

The patient receives a general anaesthetic, the laparoscope is inserted and the pelvis visualised. After a general assessment of the pelvis, the ovarian ligament is held using a pair of forceps inserted through an incision made just above the pubic hairline. Another fine needle, inserted through the abdominal wall (Figure 11.2), is used to remove the fluid from each stimulated follicle. The fluid is immediately taken to the laboratory where the embryologist looks for the egg under the microscope. If none is found the follicle is flushed with a special fluid called culture medium to see if an egg can be recovered. The flushing may have to be repeated several times.

Eggs are recovered from about 80 percent of follicles at laparoscopy. Each egg is placed in culture medium and stored in the incubator until it is ready for fertilisation.

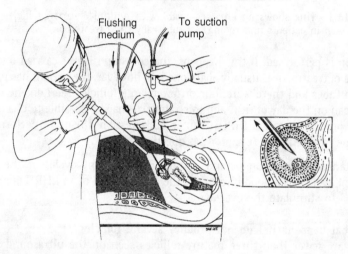

Figure 11.2 Laparoscopic egg collection. The insert shows a close-up view of the aspirating needle within the ovarian follicle.

14. How is egg collection by ultrasound performed?

Ultrasound directed egg collection is normally performed without general anaesthesia. The patient is given a tablet to relax her and an injection of an analgesic (pain relieving) and a sedative drug, either intramuscularly or into a vein on the back of the hand. The patient is awake during the procedure but drowsy because of the medication.

There are a number of ways in which ultrasound egg collection can be done (Figure 11.3) but the usual way nowadays is to use the vaginal route. In this approach, the vagina is cleansed, a vaginal ultrasound probe inserted to visualise the ovaries and a fine hollow needle is then guided through the vagina

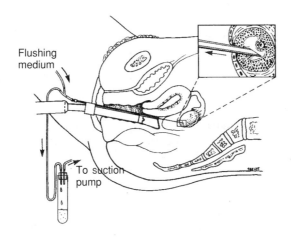

Flushing medium

To suction pump

Figure 11.3 Ultrasound directed egg collection. The insert shows a close-up view of the aspirating needle within the ovarian follicle.

into each ovary to collect the eggs. Sometimes, the ovary may be in a position that makes it impossible to reach through the vagina. In these exceptional cases, the needle may be passed either through the lower abdominal wall or through the urethra. A full bladder is necessary if these other approaches are used.

15. Is ultrasound egg collection without a general anaesthetic painful?
Most women experience only mild discomfort during the procedure but a few do complain of pain. It usually lasts only a few moments and the doctor can give another dose of analgesic drugs to relieve it. Once the procedure is over most women do not experience any pain but some may feel discomfort for a few hours, similar to that experienced after normal ovulation. This discomfort is easily relieved by a mild analgesic like paracetamol.

16. Can ultrasound egg collection be done under general anaesthesia?
It is possible but generally unnecessary. If the procedure is done under anaesthesia, the patient will have to stay in hospital as a day case. The cost of the procedure is therefore increased.

17. Is ultrasound egg collection safe?
Yes, it is a safe procedure.

Some patients notice a little blood coming from the vagina on the first day after egg collection. This is quite normal. Although there is potentially a risk of the needle puncturing a large blood vessel or the bowel or causing pelvic infection, such complications are extremely rare.

18. What are the advantages and disadvantages of ultrasound directed egg collection compared with laparoscopic egg collection?
Ultrasound directed egg collection offers a number of advantages.

First, a general anaesthetic is not needed and so it is an outpatient procedure. Second, it is safer, especially in patients with extensive adhesions caused by tubal disease or severe endometriosis, because performing a laparoscopy under these circumstances may be difficult. In some women the pelvis is so badly damaged that it is not possible to perform a laparoscopic egg collection but ultrasound guided egg collection may be feasible. Third, some patients have several attempts at IVF and it is unwise to have multiple laparoscopies and general anaesthetics.

The only advantage of laparoscopic egg collection is that the pelvis can be examined at the same time but most patients who undertake IVF will have had a laparoscopy previously as part of their infertility investigations.

19. How long does ultrasound egg collection take?
It varies, depending on the number of stimulated follicles present. The procedure usually lasts between 20-40 minutes but may require from 10 minutes to just over an hour.

20. Will egg collection damage my ovaries?
No.

Some patients worry that intensive stimulation of the ovaries will cause a premature menopause but this is something we can be very reassuring about. Only a small minority of the eggs that are lost from the ovaries as women age are lost as a result of the ovulatory process. The vast majority are lost through atresia (Chapter 1, question 3), a process which is not affected by hormones.

21. How many eggs are collected?
The number of eggs that are collected varies widely, from one to sixty! The usual number, however, is between five and fifteen. In a very small percentage of cases, no eggs can be collected at all.

22. How does fertilisation of the egg take place?
After their collection, the eggs are placed in a culture medium which nourishes them. In the meantime, a sample of the partner's sperm is prepared by a special washing technique to remove the seminal plasma and separate out the healthy sperm.

About 100,000 motile sperm are added to each egg, approximately 4-6 hours after egg collection, to allow fertilisation to take place. The exact length of time the eggs are incubated before the sperm are added depends on the maturity of the eggs.

23. When are the pre-embryos transferred?

Once fertilisation occurs, two pronuclei (one male and one female) can be seen under the microscope (Figure 11.4). The fertilised egg is called a pre-embryo and this is grown in the laboratory until 2 days after egg collection when it should be ready for transfer into the uterus. At the time of transfer, the pre-embryo is normally at the 2- to 8-cell stage (Figure 11.5).

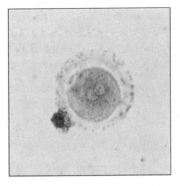

Figure 11.4   This shows a human egg with two pronuclei after it has been penetrated by the sperm but not yet fertilised.

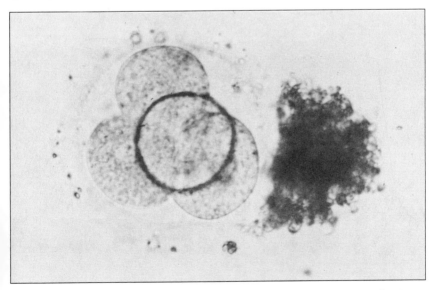

Figure 11.5   This shows a 4-cell human pre-embryo 2 days after egg collection.

24. How many pre-embryos are transferred?

The optimum number has been a matter of great debate. The reason for the debate is that the larger the number of pre-embryos transferred, the greater the chance of pregnancy in that cycle. On the other hand, the larger the number transferred, the higher is the likelihood of multiple pregnancy, including triplets and quadruplets.

Multiple pregnancies carry a high risk of miscarriage, premature birth and other obstetric complications and are associated with a higher than normal risk of long term neurological problems in the baby. As a result, the present recommendation of the Interim Licensing Authority in the United Kingdom is that a maximum of three pre-embryos be transferred. In exceptional circumstances, for example, if the patient were 40 years old, had severe endometriosis and this were her sixth attempt at IVF, four pre-embryos may be transferred. In some units, however, only two embryos are transferred.

Another reason which has encouraged the trend towards transfer of fewer pre-embryos is the development of freezing techniques. Provided they are of good quality, pre-embryos that are not transferred can be frozen and used in a subsequent cycle.

25. How is pre-embryo transfer performed?

The pre-embryos are transferred through the cervix using a fine tube (catheter, Figure 11.6). The procedure is like having a cervical smear test and takes only a few minutes. It is not at all painful.

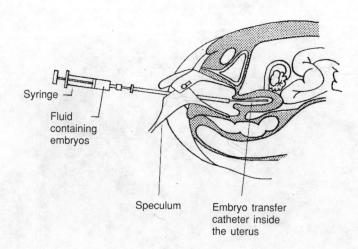

Syringe

Fluid containing embryos

Speculum

Embryo transfer catheter inside the uterus

Figure 11.6 Embryo transfer.

26. How long do I need to rest after pre-embryo transfer and can I do anything to increase my chances of pregnancy after it?
There is no evidence that resting or doing anything special increases the chances of pregnancy after pre-embryo transfer. You can resume all normal activities immediately and there is no need to take time off work. Having intercourse after pre-embryo transfer does not reduce the chances of implantation.

27. What is "luteal support" in IVF?
This involves administration of hCG or progesterone after pre-embryo transfer. There is debate concerning its value in cycles in which clomiphene and hMG are used to stimulate the ovaries but it is definitely required when LHRH analogues are used as part of the ovarian stimulation regimen.

28. Can we have intercourse during the IVF treatment cycle?
Yes.

29. When will I know if I am pregnant?
A pregnancy test is normally performed 14 days after the transfer. Since miscarriage and ectopic pregnancies can occur just as in normal pregnancies, it is advisable to have an ultrasound scan done to confirm that the pregnancy is in the uterus and is progressing normally.

30. How many IVF cycles can I have?
There is theoretically no reason why you cannot have treatment as many times as you like. Most women, however, find IVF very stressful and it is probably best to have at least 2-3 months rest between treatment cycles.

31. Are the chances of ectopic pregnancy higher after IVF?
Yes.

The reason is that many patients undergoing IVF have some degree of tubal damage. The incidence of ectopic pregnancy after IVF is about 5 percent compared with less than 1 percent in the overall population in the United Kingdom. The risk of a combined intra-uterine and ectopic pregnancy is less than one in 100.

32. What is the risk of multiple pregnancy after IVF?
The overall chance of multiple pregnancy occurring after IVF is 24 percent, or one in four pregnancies, as compared with 1 percent in spontaneous pregnancies. If two pre-embryos are transferred, the chance of twin pregnancy is about 13 percent, while if three are transferred, the incidence of twin pregnancy is about 23 percent and triplet pregnancy is about 5 percent.

When four pre-embryos are transferred over 30 percent of the pregnancies are multiple pregnancies.

The perinatal mortality rate (that is, the risk of death of a fetus between 28 weeks of pregnancy and the seventh day of life) of twins is increased threefold and of triplet and higher order pregnancy sevenfold, compared with singleton deliveries. It is largely as a result of multiple pregnancy that the overall rate of perinatal mortality after IVF (and GIFT) is three times higher than the national average.

33. What is the success rate of IVF?

There are several ways of measuring the success rate. The two that have been used most commonly are the pregnancy rate per cycle of treatment commenced and the live birth rate per cycle of treatment commenced (the "take home baby rate").

The factors that affect these outcomes are the age of the patient, the reason for infertility, the number of pre-embryos transferred in the particular cycle and the quality of the IVF treatment programme.

There is a decline in successful outcome with age, as can be seen from Table 11.1:

Table 11.1 Pregnancy rate per initiated cycle of IVF treatment at different ages.

Age (Female)	pregnancy rate per treatment cycle commenced
28 years	22%
32 years	15%
36 years	13%
40 years	9.5%

(these are the results of a recent analysis we and our colleagues have made of more than 5,000 treatment cycles of IVF).

Miscarriage rates rise with maternal age so the "take-home baby rate" falls even more than these figures indicate.

With regard to the causes of infertility, the success rates are little different, except for couples with male infertility or multiple causes of infertility, in which cases the chances of pregnancy fall significantly.

With regard to the number of pre-embryos transferred, the 1990 report of the Interim Licensing Authority of the United Kingdom indicated that the overall pregnancy rates in 1988 were 9.6 percent, 14.2 percent, 25.2 percent and 23.4 percent after one, two, three and four pre-embryos were transferred.

That report also indicated that, in the United Kingdom, large centres (that is, those undertaking more than 400 treatment cycles per year) had better overall results than smaller units, especially those undertaking fewer than 100 cycles per year.

34. What are my chances of success if I have more than one attempt at IVF?

Perhaps the best measures of success in IVF are the **cumulative conception** and **cumulative live birth rates**. These describe the likelihood of a person becoming pregnant or having a live birth after a specified number of cycles of treatment. For example, a cumulative conception rate of 40 percent after three cycles means that 40 percent of women will have become pregnant after three cycles of treatment. Use of cumulative rates allows one to make direct comparisons of different methods of treatment and are especially important nowadays because many patients undergo repeated attempts at IVF.

The most important factor affecting these rates is again the age of the patient. In Figure 11.7 you can see that the cumulative rate of conception increases as the number of cycles of treatment increases. There is, however, a fall in the pregnancy rate as women age.

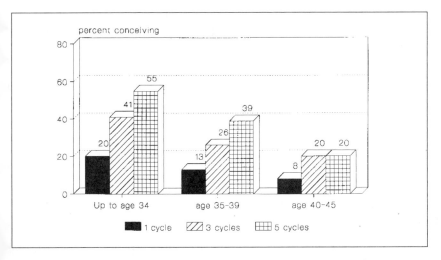

Figure 11.7 Cumulative conception rate in IVF, related to the woman's age.

The conception rate in women aged 40-45 after five cycles of treatment is the same as in women up to the age of 34 after one cycle.

In Figure 11.8 you can see the effect of age on the cumulative live birth rate — that is the "take-home baby rate".

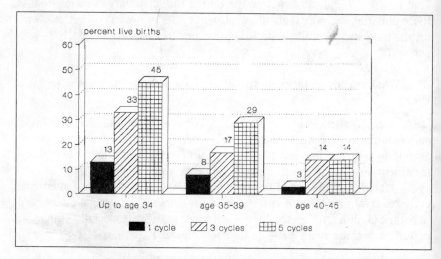

Figure 11.8 Cumulative live birth rate in IVF, related to the woman's age.

While the take-home baby rate is almost 50 percent after five cycles of treatment in the youngest group of women, the realistic chances of success for a woman over the age of 40 are very disappointing indeed. In our opinion, women over the age of 40 should consider very carefully before undertaking any of the techniques of assisted fertility.

35. How much does IVF cost?
The cost varies from one country to another.

In the United Kingdom, the usual cost ranges from £1,000 to £2,000 for each treatment cycle, excluding the cost of drugs.

When comparing costs it is important to determine exactly what is included in the fees.

36. Does IVF increase the chance of an abnormal baby?
No.

There is an underlying risk of congenital abnormality in all pregnancies of about 2-3 percent and while IVF does not protect against having abnormal babies, it does not increase the risk either. Thousands of babies have now been born worldwide as an result of IVF and no increase in the incidence of fetal abnormality has been found.

37. Can I select the sex of my baby in IVF?

Sex selection using IVF was not possible until very recently. Research has now shown that it is possible, by removing one cell from the developing pre-embryo, to test to see if it carries the male (Y) chromosome. The technique is not yet widely available. When it is perfected it will open the door to the prevention of sex-linked hereditary diseases. Since these disorders are only manifest in males, those with such disorders could undergo IVF and select only female pre-embryos for transfer.

On the other hand, IVF should never be used to select the sex of a baby unless there is a medical reason to do so.

38. Can IVF be used to prevent congenital abnormalities?

The use of IVF to prevent congenital abnormalities is very much in its infancy but it is at the forefront of today's research. The principle is to determine, before transfer, whether the pre-embryo contains the gene responsible for a particular condition. If it does, that pre-embryo is not transferred. This technique, which requires analysis of the genetic material (the DNA) from a single cell that has been removed from the pre-embryo, is very much at the research stage. There is no doubt, however, that in the next few years, medical advances will allow an increasing number of diseases to be prevented by IVF techniques.

39. Can you get IVF on the National Health Service?

There are only two IVF units in the United Kingdom that are fully funded by the National Health Service (NHS). They are in Manchester and Cardiff. Naturally these units can only accept patients from their own areas.

There are seventeen IVF units which are linked to the National Health Service. In these units, treatment of NHS patients is subsidised by the fees paid by the fully paying private patients.

The vast majority of patients, however, who have IVF do so in one of the twenty-three private IVF clinics in the United Kingdom.

40. What is embryo freezing (cryopreservation)?

This is a procedure in which pre-embryos, in excess of those transferred in the cycle in which the eggs were collected, are frozen and stored so they can be transferred in a subsequent cycle. Only good quality pre-embryos can survive the freezing procedure.

41. What is the success rate of embryo freezing?

It largely depends on the stage at which the pre-embryo is frozen. At present, the highest success rates are obtained when it is frozen at the pronucleate stage and roughly 80 percent of these pre-embryos survive the freezing and thawing process. The chance of frozen pre-embryos leading to pregnancy is more or less the same as for fresh pre-embryos. No increased risk of abnormal babies has been found with the use of frozen pre-embryos.

42. What is intra-vaginal culture?

This is a recently developed variation of IVF, which hopefully will cut the cost of IVF.

After the eggs have been collected, they are placed with the partner's sperm in a small tube containing culture medium. The tube is sealed, placed in the patient's vagina and held in place by a contraceptive cap. The cap and tube are removed 24-48 hours later and the contents inspected for evidence of fertilisation. The resulting pre-embryos are transferred into the uterus by the standard method.

43. What is transport IVF?

Another development which aims to cut the costs of IVF, in this case, quite dramatically. It involves several satellite hospitals or clinics being able to use the facilities of a centrally placed embryology unit.

The woman remains under the supervision and treatment of her local hospital or clinic where the ovarian stimulation and egg collection are performed. On the day of egg collection her partner provides a sample of his sperm at the specialist centre. He is given a pre-warmed incubator which is plugged into the cigarette lighter socket in the car dashboard. He drives to the local hospital where the eggs are collected and placed in the incubator and he then returns to the specialist centre. Here, his sperm are used to fertilise the eggs, using standard techniques. Two days later the woman is called to the centre for a standard pre-embryo transfer.

44. What is egg donation?

Egg donation is the procedure in which an infertile patient who cannot produce her own eggs receives a donated egg from another woman. The sperm that are used to fertilise the egg come from the partner of the infertile patient.

45. Who needs donated eggs?

Some women are infertile because they cannot produce eggs. This happens either because their ovaries have never developed properly, or because their ovaries have stopped functioning as a result of premature menopause or damage by infection, surgery or chemotherapy. For these women, donated eggs offer hope of pregnancy.

The second group of women who will benefit from egg donation are those who are carriers of sex-linked genetic diseases, such as haemophilia or Duchenne muscular dystrophy.

46. Where do donated eggs come from?
There are two types of donors.

They may be volunteers who have completed their family and agree to have eggs collected at a sterilisation procedure or women who undergo ovarian stimulation and egg collection purely to donate eggs to others. The other group of donors are patients undergoing IVF treatment who produce a large number of eggs, in excess of what is needed for themselves.

Any decision to donate eggs has to be preceded by very careful discussion; it is not a decision that would ever be taken without the well informed consent of the donor.

47. Is egg donation anonymous?
Although it is possible for patients to bring donors, most IVF programmes operate egg donation programmes on an anonymous basis only, so that the recipient and donor are not told who the other party was. In this sense the programme operates much the same way as sperm banks.

48. Will the baby look like me?
Half of the baby's genes will come from your partner and half from the egg donor. Although most IVF programmes try to find a donor who matches the recipient's physical characteristics, in practice, the supply of eggs is so limited that matching is limited too.

49. What does the treatment involve for the recipient of egg donation?
If the recipient has stopped menstruating completely and does not produce the normal amounts of female hormones, she is given hormone treatment in the form of oestrogen tablets or patches and progesterone injections or suppositories to prepare the lining of the uterus for pregnancy. In the first month of therapy, several blood tests may be needed to ensure that her hormone levels are normal. If the recipient has normal menstrual cycles, hormone tablets may be given to adjust her cycle and delay her period.

50. What happens in the laboratory?
In the laboratory, the donated egg is mixed with a sample of the recipient's partner's sperm. The rest of the procedure is the same as for normal IVF.

51. How is the pre-embryo transfer performed?
Exactly the same way as in normal IVF.

52. What is the success rate for ovum donation?
In 1988, a total of 122 patients were treated by ovum donation in the United Kingdom; twenty pregnancies resulted, giving a pregnancy rate of 15 percent per cycle. These results compare favourably with standard IVF.

53. What about freezing eggs?
Unfortunately attempts so far to preserve eggs by freezing have been largely unsuccessful but research is underway to find ways of improving the technique.

54. What is "micromanipulation"?
The egg has a tough outer coating called the zona pellucida, which is thought to be the main barrier to the penetration of sperm. In cases of male factor infertility the ability of sperm to penetrate the zona may be reduced. Several micromanipulation procedures have been devised to help the sperm pass through the zona.

At present, these methods are very much at the research stage but are being tried in cases of severe male infertility when conventional IVF has failed. A micromanipulator is used, which magnifies the egg many times and permits the various intricate procedures to be performed. These involve stripping the egg of its outer cells, positioning it on a holding pipette and then either making a small opening in the zona pellucida (so the sperm can pass through) or directly injecting the sperm through the zona pellucida.

12

GIFT AND OTHER METHODS OF ASSISTED FERTILITY

1. What is GIFT? +ZIFT + TEST (see late)

GIFT stands for gamete intra-fallopian transfer.

It is an alternative treatment to IVF for women who have patent (that is, not blocked) fallopian tubes. The first few steps are similar to those used for IVF, namely, ovarian stimulation with drugs, monitoring of follicular growth, administration of hCG to induce final maturation of the eggs and egg collection (usually by laparoscopy).

Once the eggs have been collected, they are placed in a laboratory dish, observed under a microscope and their maturity noted. Sperm and eggs are then drawn separately into a fine catheter and transferred into the patient's fallopian tubes (Figure 12.1).

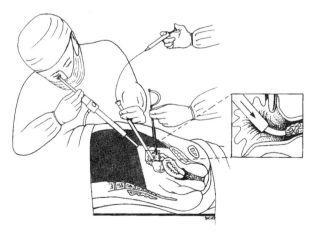

Figure 12.1 A GIFT procedure being performed. The insert shows a close-up of the catheter within the fallopian tube. The sperms and eggs are gently flushed into the fallopian tube.

The main difference between GIFT and IVF is that, in GIFT, fertilisation occurs within the fallopian tube and not in the laboratory. The resulting pre-embryo, or pre-embryos, then move down the fallopian tubes into the uterus where they implant.

However, because fertilisation is not directly observed in the GIFT procedure, one cannot be certain that fertilisation has occurred unless pregnancy follows.

2. What types of infertility patients are suitable for GIFT?
The indications for GIFT are the same as those for IVF except that the patient **must** have patent fallopian tubes. Moreover the procedure involves laparoscopy and, therefore, general anaesthesia.

3. What drugs are given to stimulate the ovaries?
The drug regimens used for GIFT are identical to those for IVF (Chapter 11, question 5).

4. How is follicular growth monitored?
Monitoring of follicular growth is achieved in an identical fashion to that used for IVF (Chapter 11, question 9).

5. Are all the eggs collected transferred into the fallopian tubes?
Not necessarily.

The current recommendation by the Interim Licensing Authority of the United Kingdom is that no more than three eggs should be transferred in any one cycle, unless there are exceptional clinical circumstances, when four may be replaced.

6. What happens to the excess eggs?
They are generally fertilised with your partner's sperm as a test of fertilisation; the resulting pre-embryos can then be frozen to be used in a subsequent cycle for transfer into your uterus, as in IVF programmes. Excess eggs can also be donated to someone else (Chapter 11, question 44).

Sometimes, a patient is scheduled for GIFT but her tubes are unexpectedly found to be abnormal at the time of laparoscopy. In such cases, the eggs can be collected and the procedure converted to IVF, that is, the eggs are fertilised with the partner's sperm and the pre-embryo(s) transferred into the uterus 2 days later.

7. How long does the GIFT procedure take?
This depends on the number of follicles present and can vary considerably but most GIFT procedures last between 30-60 minutes.

8.   What is the success rate of GIFT?
The overall pregnancy rate per treatment cycle for GIFT is approximately 21 percent.

9.   What are the complications associated with the GIFT procedure?
They are similar to those in IVF when laparoscopic egg collection is used.

Apart from anaesthetic complications, the laparoscope can rarely puncture bowel, bladder or blood vessels. In the hands of experienced surgeons, however, such complications are very rare but if they do inadvertently occur, they are, of course, immediately corrected surgically. The usual side effects are drowsiness and nausea for a few hours and sore throat caused by the tube being passed down the throat during anaesthesia. Some patients may have slight abdominal or chest discomfort for a few days because of the gas that has been used to distend the abdominal cavity.

Most patients can leave the hospital a few hours after the GIFT procedure and can return to work within a day or two.

10.   Can we have intercourse during the GIFT cycle?
Yes.

11.   Is the risk of multiple pregnancy increased with GIFT?
Yes.

The risk of multiple pregnancy is increased with GIFT just as it is with IVF.

The overall multiple pregnancy rate in GIFT is about 21 percent and is directly related to the number of eggs transferred. In the 1990 report of the Interim Licensing Authority of the United Kingdom, it was noted that when five or more eggs were replaced, although there was no significant increase in the pregnancy rate compared to when fewer eggs were transferred, the rate of multiple pregnancy rose to 31 percent.

The complications of multiple birth are the same as they are for IVF (Chapter 11, question 32).

12.   Does GIFT increase the chances of fetal abnormality?
There is no increased risk of fetal abnormality after GIFT.

13.   What is DIPI?
DIPI stands for direct intra-peritoneal insemination.

It involves four steps. The first three are similar to IVF, that is, stimulation of the ovaries with drugs, monitoring of the growth of the follicles and administration of an hCG injection to cause egg maturation when the follicles are judged to be ripe.

The final step is to inject a washed, sample of semen through the top of the vagina into the abdominal cavity immediately behind the uterus (the Pouch of Douglas, Figure 12.2) 36 hours after the injection of hCG. This can either be done "blindly" or else under ultrasound guidance. The procedure is quick and is performed as an out-patient procedure. The patient can go home immediately.

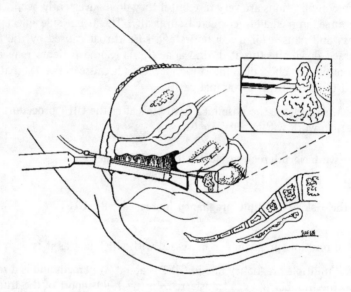

Figure 12.2 Direct intra-peritoreal insemination (DIPI). This shows a sample of washed sperm being injected into the Pouch of Douglas at the time of presumed ovulation.

14. Which patients would benefit from DIPI?

DIPI may be used for patients with a variety of infertility problems, including unexplained infertility, cervical mucus hostility, low sperm counts and failed donor insemination. It is, however, not a very successful method and generally should be considered only if more sophisticated techniques are not available. One situation where it may be useful is in patients with patent fallopian tubes who are undergoing IVF in whom ovulation has inadvertently occurred before egg collection.

15. What is the success rate of DIPI?

DIPI is not a very successful technique and when all the published results are pooled, the pregnancy rate is roughly 10 percent per treatment cycle. Another problem is that if more than four large follicles develop as a result of ovarian stimulation, the possibility of high order multiple pregnancy (triplets or more) makes DIPI inappropriate and the patient's treatment must be converted to another procedure such as POST, IVF or GIFT.

16. What does POST stand for?

POST stands for peritoneal oocyte and sperm transfer.

It consists of five steps. The first four are the same as in IVF, namely, stimulation of the ovaries with drugs, monitoring of follicular growth, administration of hCG to allow final maturation of the eggs and ultrasound directed egg recovery. The last step involves transferring a maximum of three or four eggs together with a prepared sample of washed sperm into the Pouch of Douglas close to the fallopian tubes (Figure 12.3).

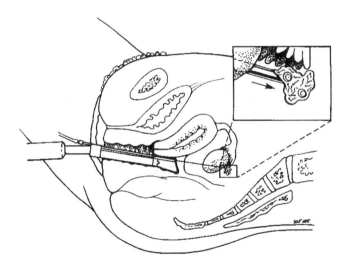

Figure 12.3 Peritoneal occyte sperm transfer (POST). In this procedure both eggs and sperm are injected into the Pouch of Douglas close to the opening of the fallopian tube.

The main advantage of POST is that the laboratory work involved with IVF and embryo transfer are unnecessary. Unlike GIFT, no laparoscopy or general anaesthesia is needed either.

17. What types of patients are suitable for POST?

POST can only be performed if the fallopian tubes are patent. The major indications for which it has been used are in patients with unexplained infertility, in those where donor insemination has failed and in patients with sperm mucus antibody problems.

18. What is the success rate of POST?

The overall pregnancy rate is about 25 percent per cycle of treatment.

19. Is there an increased risk of fetal abnormality with POST?

There is no evidence that the risk of fetal abnormality is increased when POST is used.

20. What do ZIFT, PROST, TET, and TEST stand for?

ZIFT stands for zygote intra-fallopian tube transfer. PROST stands for pronuclear stage tubal transfer. TET is short for tubal embryo transfer while TEST is tubal embryo stage transfer.

21. What is the difference between these techniques?

ZIFT and PROST are acronyms for the same procedure and TET and TEST refer to the same procedure.

In all four procedures, ovarian stimulation with drugs, monitoring of follicular growth, timed administration of hCG injection, ultrasound directed egg collection and in-vitro fertilisation of the eggs with sperm in the laboratory are carried out as in IVF.

In the case of ZIFT and PROST, fertilised eggs are transferred into the fallopian tubes at laparoscopy when the pronuclei are seen 18 hours after insemination. In the case of TET or TEST transfer of the fertilised eggs into the fallopian tubes is also performed by laparoscopy but the procedure is delayed until the pre-embryo has divided into two or more cells.

22. When are these procedures used?

Although, in theory, both of these assisted conception techniques can be used for all of the cases suitable for GIFT, in practice, they have mainly been advocated for patients with male infertility.

Their main advantage is that the eggs are exposed to high concentrations of motile sperm, increasing the chances of fertilisation. The fertilisation can be directly observed, unlike in the GIFT technique. Compared with IVF, the theoretical advantage is that the fertilised egg is allowed to develop in the fallopian tube instead of uterus and so mimic the natural situation more closely.

23. How successful are these procedures?

It is difficult to compare results because so far there have been very few scientific studies using these techniques and they have contained few cases. So far, pregnancy rates have varied from 17-37 percent per cycle.

24. What is DOT?

DOT stands for direct oocyte transfer.

In this technique, ovarian stimulation with drugs, monitoring of follicular growth, timed hCG administration, and ultrasound directed egg collection are all carried out as in IVF.

After the eggs have been collected, they are incubated in culture medium for a few hours and sperm are then added. When sperm are seen to be bound to the egg, a maximum of three eggs are transferred into the uterus, using the technique of conventional embryo transfer, as in IVF. This technique is still in its infancy and only a few pregnancies have been reported using it.

25. What is TUFT?

TUFT stands for trans-uterine fallopian transfer.

In this procedure a fine tube is passed into the fallopian tube through the vagina and uterus. The device used consists of a flexible outer tube, which is kept straight with an inner metal piece, and a soft open ended inner catheter (Figure 12.4). The outer tube is passed into the uterine cavity and the inner metal piece then removed so that the outer cannula regains its natural,

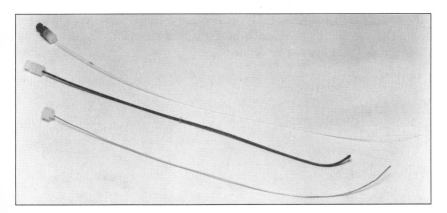

Figure 12.4 Components of the instrument used for catheterising the fallopian tube through the uterine cavity.

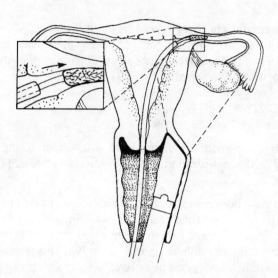

Figure 12.5 This photograph shows catheterisation of the fallopian tube through the uterine cavity. The procedure is being performed under ultrasound guidance.

laterally directed, curve. The outer tube is then advanced slowly under ultrasound guidance towards the fallopian tube (Figure 12.5). The catheter is then threaded through the outer tube into the fallopian tube.

Using this technique, pre-embryos have been transferred into the fallopian tube and pregnancies achieved. The main advantage of TUFT compared with GIFT or ZIFT is that laparoscopy is not necessary. This is, however, still a very new technique and more research needs to be done before its place in the treatment of infertility can be defined.

13

THE CERVICAL FACTOR, UTERINE
PROBLEMS AND UNEXPLAINED
INFERTILITY

**1.   My uterus is tilted backwards. One of my friends had an operation to
make her uterus tilt forwards. Is this a good treatment for infertility?**
Twenty percent of women have a uterus that is tilted backwards, that is to say,
a retroverted uterus (Figure 13.1). This is a normal variation, just as some of
us are left handed.

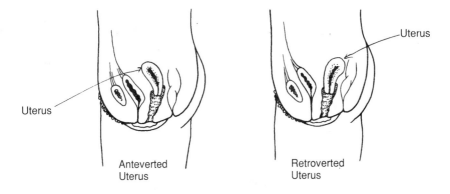

Figure 13.1   An anteverted uterus points forwards while a retroverted uterus points
backwards.

A retroverted uterus does not by itself cause infertility. For a woman with a
normal, mobile, retroverted uterus, there is no advantage in having an operation (called **ventrosuspension**) to antevert the uterus, that is, to make it
tilt forwards. In such cases, ventrosuspension does not cure the infertility. It
often fails to maintain the uterus in a forward position and may, occasionally,
even contribute to infertility because it can lead to the formation of adhesions
that kink the fallopian tubes.

135

There are some women, however, with endometriosis or pelvic adhesions in whom the uterus becomes stuck backwards as part of the disease process. In these cases the uterus is fixed and can be distinguished from normal retroversion at pelvic examination. In these cases, ventrosuspension may sometimes be usefully performed as part of a conservative operation for the treatment of endometriosis.

2. Do fibroids cause infertility?

Fibroids are benign growths of muscle which appear in the wall of the uterus. They are very common and it has been estimated that one in three women at the age of 40 have some fibroids in the uterus. Most fibroids, however, are very small, do not cause any symptoms and are never detected.

In a minority of women, fibroids can lead to heavy or abnormal menstrual bleeding. Rarely, large fibroids distort the uterine cavity and so cause miscarriage or infertility by preventing the pre-embryo from implanting.

3. Does removing fibroids improve fertility?

Many women with fibroids conceive without difficulty, have uneventful pregnancies and deliver normally. If an asymptomatic fibroid is found during physical examination in an infertile patient, it is important to look for other causes of infertility and treat those other problems first.

Surgical removal of asymptomatic fibroids is only necessary if the fibroids are very large or if there are no other causes of infertility detected and the position of the fibroid is such that it may distort the uterine cavity (Figure 13.2).

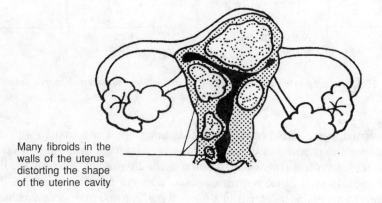

Many fibroids in the walls of the uterus distorting the shape of the uterine cavity

Figure 13.2 Fibroids and infertility.

4.   I have been told that some women cannot get pregnant because their uteruses have abnormal shapes. Can you tell me more about this?

Some women are born with abnormal development of the uterus. The abnormalities include a double uterus, a uterus with a septum, a heart shaped uterus, a uterus which does not communicate with the vagina or even complete absence of the uterus (Figure 13.3).

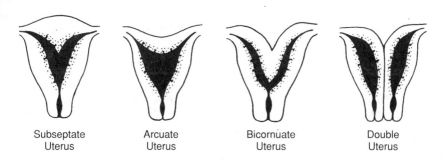

| Subseptate Uterus | Arcuate Uterus | Bicornuate Uterus | Double Uterus |

Figure 13.3   A diagrammatic representation of some abnormal uterine shapes.

Most women with a double or heart-shaped uterus have no difficulty conceiving and have uneventful pregnancies. However, there is a higher risk of late miscarriage. Rarely, some abnormally shaped uteruses may be associated with infertility and, in exceptional cases, surgery may be advised to correct these abnormalities.

5.   Does scarring of the uterine cavity after a D & C cause infertility? Is this common and what is the treatment?

In very rare cases, excessive scraping of the uterus, for example, after a termination of pregnancy or miscarriage, may lead to the formation of adhesions within the uterine cavity. These adhesions can cause the walls of the uterus to become completely or partially stuck together (Ashermann's syndrome). Treatment involves dividing the adhesions.

The procedure is rather like a D & C and may be performed under direct vision through a hysteroscope (Chapter 5, question 42), which is a telescope inserted into the uterus. Once the adhesions are divided, the gynaecologist may insert an IUCD or catheter into the uterus for a few weeks so that the walls of the uterus do not get stuck together again. Antibiotics and hormones are usually given to prevent infection and to encourage the endometrial lining to re-grow.

6. What is cervical mucus and what is its function?
Cervical mucus is a jelly-like substance produced by tiny glands in the cervical canal. It acts like a plug in the cervix. It has a number of functions. First, it helps to prevent bacteria from entering the uterine cavity. Second, its composition changes during the different phases of the menstrual cycle so that sperm can penetrate it easily around the time of ovulation but not at other times (which is why a post-coital test (Chapter 5, question 26) must be accurately timed).

Once sperm penetrate the cervical mucus, they can survive there for at least 72 hours. The mucus therefore acts as a sperm reservoir and helps pregnancy to occur even if intercourse had not occurred precisely at the time of ovulation.

At the beginning of the menstrual cycle, the cervical mucus is very scanty. As the amount of oestrogen produced by the developing ovarian follicle increases, the mucus becomes more watery and copious and just before ovulation occurs, it can be so much as to resemble a watery vaginal discharge. Its consistency at this time is like raw egg white. Once ovulation occurs, the mucus becomes thicker and more sticky because of the action of progesterone and sperm can no longer get through.

7. I have been told that my cervical mucus has antibodies which prevent my husband's sperm from passing through. What does this mean?
Antibodies are substances produced by the body's defence mechanism in response to foreign material. These antibodies protect the body from infection by bacteria and viruses.

It has been found that some infertile women produce antibodies against sperm and it has been suggested that this could be a cause of infertility. The problem is made a little more complicated because such antibodies have also been found in fertile and even pregnant women!

8. Can a man produce antibodies against sperm?
Yes. It has also been found that some men, who have sluggish sperm, or sperm that do not penetrate cervical mucus well, produce anti-sperm antibodies.

In order to find out if antibodies are produced by the woman or her partner, a cross challenge test can be performed. In this test, some of the woman's mucus is mixed with sperm from a donor, while her partner's sperm are mixed with donor mucus. Both samples are examined under the microscope and so it can be determined whether the problem lies in the sperm or the mucus.

9. What is the treatment for infertility caused by antibody formation?
A lot of different treatments have been tried.

They include asking the woman's partner to wear a condom for 6 months whenever they have intercourse so that the sperm and cervical mucus do not come into contact, or giving steroid or immunosuppressive drugs to prevent antibody formation.

The problem is that if the couple is going to use a condom whenever they have sex, they are not going to get pregnant and there is no good evidence that the infertility will be cured after 6 months. Immunosuppressive drugs have been reported by some clinics to be successful but others have found that they are of no value. One problem with such drugs is the high incidence of side effects associated with their use. This is particularly the case with steroid treatment because the drugs are given in very large doses.

Another treatment that is often used is sperm washing and intra-uterine insemination. The effectiveness of this method has also been questioned because if the woman is producing antibodies, these may be present in the uterine cavity and fallopian tubes as well and simply by-passing the cervical mucus may not be good enough.

The most effective treatment is in-vitro fertilisation because even if the woman produces antibodies, this does not seem to prevent fertilisation of the egg in the laboratory. The final possibility is to use donor sperm.

10. If the cervical mucus is poor, can treatment with oestrogens improve it?

The most common reasons for finding poor cervical mucus are failure of ovulation or a wrongly timed test but it can also be caused by chronic inflammation or by a previous cone biopsy of the cervix.

Provided ovulation is confirmed, the first thing to do if poor cervical mucus is found is to ensure that the mucus test was performed at the correct time. The most reliable way is to have serial ultrasound scans to monitor the growth of the ovarian follicle and to check the mucus just before ovulation.

It has been suggested that if the cervical mucus is scanty and thick even when checked at the correct time, giving oestrogens may help. Unfortunately, it has been found that the administration of oestrogens often disturbs ovulation.

Intra-uterine insemination is probably a better solution for such cases. In this technique, a fine catheter is passed into the uterus through the cervix and a sample of washed, prepared sperm injected into the uterine cavity (Figure 13.4). Unwashed semen should not be used because of the risk of infection, and also of severe cramps which are caused by prostaglandins, a normal constituent of semen.

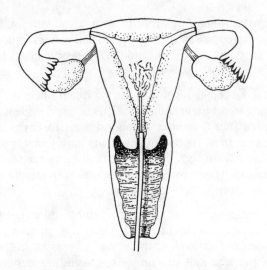

Figure 13.4 Intra-uterine insemination. A fine catheter is threaded into the uterine cavity and a sample of washed sperm are injected through it.

11. What is "unexplained infertility"?

Unexplained infertility is said to be present if no cause has been found after both partners have been fully investigated.

The minimum investigations that should have been performed before such a diagnosis is made include a normal semen analysis, demonstration of normal ovulation, as shown by blood tests and ultrasound scans (not just a basal body temperature chart), a normal pelvis with patent tubes demonstrated at laparoscopy (a hysterosalpingogram is not sufficient) and a normal post-coital test.

12. What proportion of infertile couples have unexplained infertility?

It depends entirely on how detailed the investigations have been. For example, if laparoscopy is omitted, some clinics report a figure as high as 25 percent because many cases of endometriosis and pelvic adhesions will be missed.

Most centres find that 5-15 percent of infertile couples have this diagnosis made after complete investigations have been performed. Of course, the definition of "completeness" changes all the time because of research. For example, we now consider a measurement of serum LH in the follicular phase to be part of the routine investigation of an infertile couple (Chapter 7, question 36).

13. What is the treatment of unexplained infertility?

A host of treatments have been tried.

As a background to the assessment of any therapy proposed for unexplained infertility, it must be appreciated that some of these couples get pregnant without any treatment at all. Many of these couples have reduced fertility and perhaps need a little longer than average to conceive. However, since fertility in women falls with age and, as it is known from plotting cumulative conception rates for patients with unexplained infertility that the longer the duration of infertility the less the likelihood of a spontaneous pregnancy, it is reasonable to propose some active form of treatment if the unexplained infertility has lasted for more than 3 years. The length of time, of course, also depends on the age of the woman and the older she is, the shorter the duration of unexplained infertility before treatment is advised.

The most successful treatments at present appear to be super-ovulation combined with monitoring of ovulation and intra-uterine insemination, in-vitro fertilisation, GIFT and the other newer assisted reproductive techniques, described in Chapter 12.

14

MALE INFERTILITY

1.   What causes male infertility?

Male infertility exists if the man's semen contains no sperm (azoospermia), too few sperm (oligospermia), poor quality sperm or a high percentage of abnormal sperm. Important factors include the presence of sperm antibodies and infections. Infertility can also be caused by some sexual problem so that the man fails to impregnate his partner or ejaculate his semen into the vagina.

2.   What causes a complete absence of sperm in the semen?

This occurs either because no sperm are produced by the testes or because they are not ejaculated during orgasm. In turn, the latter may arise because the tubes leading from the testes to the seminal vesicles are blocked or the muscles that pump semen through the penis are not functioning properly.

Complete failure of the testes to produce sperm is, fortunately, rare and accounts for less than 5 percent of cases of male infertility. It arises either because the pituitary gland does not produce the necessary hormones to stimulate the testes (**male hypogonadotrophic hypogonadism**) or because the testes are unable to respond to these hormones (**primary testicular failure**). Primary testicular failure may be caused by genetic defects, undescended testes, physical injury to the testes or mumps (if it occurs after puberty). Very often the reason for primary testicular failure in a particular man is not known.

Blockage of the tubes leading from the testes to the urethra may sometimes be genetic or caused by injury, but is usually because of infection leading to scarring of the tubes.

In less than 1 percent of men the muscles that pump semen through the penis do not act in a coordinated way so that the sperm enter the bladder and mix with the urine instead of getting into the vagina. This condition, called **retrograde ejaculation**, may be caused by certain drugs, such as guanethidine (used to treat high blood pressure), nerve damage (for example due to diabetes mellitus) or it may follow an operation to remove the prostate gland.

3.   Is there any treatment for azoospermia?
It depends on the cause.

Infertility caused by primary testicular failure cannot be treated except by donor insemination. On the other hand, male hypogonadotrophic hypogonadism is easily treated. It can be distinguished from primary testicular failure by the presence of small soft testicles with a low blood FSH level — unlike primary testicular failure where the testes are usually firm and the FSH level is elevated.

Treatment of hypogonadotrophic hypogonadism consists of taking bromocriptine if the blood prolactin level is high, or, if it is not, having hMG and hCG injections to stimulate the testes or using an LHRH pump to stimulate the patient's own pituitary to produce FSH and LH.

Retrograde ejaculation is usually treated by recovering live sperm from the urine after masturbation and performing artificial insemination.

4.   If I have a low sperm count, does this mean I am not virile?
No.

This is a very common misconception. There is no relationship between sperm count and virility. There are very virile men who have a low sperm count and there are men who are impotent but who have completely normal sperm counts.

5.   What is a varicocele and does it cause infertility?
A varicocele is a collection of dilated, tortuous veins in the scrotum around the testicles, somewhat like varicose veins. It is more common on the left side. It occurs in about 10 percent of men and generally produces no discomfort. It can be detected as a soft swelling above the testicle when the man is examined standing up.

The most widely accepted reason to explain a relationship between varicocele and male infertility is that the sluggish blood flow through the swollen veins raises the scrotal temperature (testicular temperature is normally about 1°C lower than the body's core temperature). There is no proof, however, of this explanation. Indeed, many doctors now doubt that varicocele have very much to do with male infertility. They point out that most infertile men do not have varicocele while the majority of men with varicocele have normal sperm production.

6. Does surgery for varicocele improve fertility?
This is controversial. There are many infertility specialists who believe that surgical correction of the varicocele improves the sperm count and motility in infertile men (surgery in these cases involves tying off the abnormal vessels through a small incision made in the groin). Other equally experienced specialists believe that surgery for varicocele does not improve male infertility at all.

In our opinion, the place for operation is in the man with a varicocele who has a sperm count that shows both an impairment of motility as well as reduced number of sperm and who has no other explanation for infertility.

7. Can undescended testes cause infertility in later life?
Yes. This is one of the reasons why doctors recommend that the operation to bring the testes into the scrotum is done when the child is very young (about the age of 6). But it must be accepted that sometimes the reason the testicle has not descended into the scrotum is because it was abnormal in the first place and so surgically re-positioning it may not necessarily prevent subsequent infertility.

8. Does masturbation or excessive intercourse cause infertility?
No.

9. Does tight underwear cause infertility? Does wearing loose clothing and having cold showers improve the sperm count? What other general advice would you give?
Unlike the situation in women, in which specific treatments exist for specific causes of infertility, most methods of treating male infertility are poorly established. Since only one sperm is needed to produce a baby, it may be possible even for men with very low sperm counts to produce a baby eventually, although the chances are much lower than normal. Because male infertility itself is not very well understood, many of the treatments used are empirical.

It is a good idea to maintain a normal body weight and have moderate regular exercise. There is no proof that bathing the scrotum daily in cold water improves the sperm count. On the other hand, wearing loose fitting underpants does no harm and you may feel that you are doing everything possible to help nature — which arranged for sperm production to take place in an environment that is a little cooler than body temperature. Certainly, it would seem a good idea to avoid very hot baths and saunas.

With regard to smoking, drinking and drugs, there is good evidence that they can adversely affect sperm production. Smoking reduces sperm counts and motility so it is a good idea to give up smoking or, at least, reduce it to the absolute minimum. Drugs such as marijuana also diminish sperm production.

With regard to alcohol, excessive drinking impairs sperm production and may diminish sexual performance. As Shakespeare observed "It . . . provokes the desire but it takes away the performance" (Macbeth, II:3). In fact, impotence is a problem associated with chronic alcoholism. There are no exact limits as to the amount of alcohol consumption permitted if there is a male infertility problem. However, it is reasonable to avoid more than three to four pints of beer a day or their equivalent in other spirits.

10. Does mumps cause infertility?
If mumps occurs after puberty, it affects the testes (mumps orchitis) in 20 percent of cases. If both are affected, sperm production is usually reduced.

11. What other infections cause infertility?
A number of infections can cause infertility. They include sexually transmitted diseases such as gonorrhoea, clamydiae and mycoplasma as well as systemic infections such as tuberculosis. Severe infections with certain bacteria can cause blockage of the tubes that transport sperm from the testes. More commonly, they reduce sperm production and motility.

12. Do antibiotics help infertility in men?
Only if the infertility is associated with infection.

The best results are obtained if the actual bacteria are isolated, antibiotic sensitivities identified and the precise antibiotics prescribed. Very often the precise organisms cannot be isolated and infection is suspected because the number of white blood cells in the semen is increased. In such cases, most doctors would prescribe antibiotics on the basis that there may be something to be gained and nothing to lose. Both partners should be treated and the antibiotic usually chosen is one that is concentrated in the secretions of the genital tract, such as doxycycline.

13. Does giving male hormones improve fertility?
If there is proven hormone deficiency, giving male hormones will improve fertility. If there is no proven hormone deficiency (the vast majority of cases), the response to gonadotrophin therapy is disappointing and such treatment must be considered purely empirical. With regard to mesterolone (an androgen) the results are controversial, some doctors reporting beneficial effects on the sperm count and sperm motility while others have found no difference compared with treatment with a placebo.

Except in cases of proven hormone deficiency, we are not convinced that hormone treatments are effective for treating male infertility.

14. Does taking fertility pills improve male fertility?

Both clomiphene citrate and tamoxifen have been used to try to improve the sperm count. Although some doctors have found these drugs effective, there is no good evidence that they improve male fertility. We do not use them.

15. What is artificial insemination with the husband's semen and how is it done?

Artificial insemination with the husband's semen (AIH) is a procedure whereby the husband's sperm are introduced into the wife's genital tract artificially instead of by natural intercourse.

Insemination can be either into the cervix or into the uterus itself. In the first procedure, the patient lies on an examination table with her knees bent, a speculum is passed into the vagina and the cervix is visualised. The semen, which will have been obtained by masturbation, is introduced directly into the cervix and vagina. In the second method of AIH, the patient adopts a similar position, a fine plastic tube is inserted into the uterus and sperm are injected directly into the uterine cavity. This procedure is called **intra-uterine insemination (IUI)**.

16. What is the split ejaculate method of AIH?

At the time of ejaculation, most of the sperm are released in the initial part of the ejaculate while the rest of the seminal fluid tends to contain many fewer sperm. The split ejaculate method is designed to separate the first part of the ejaculate from the rest so that a more concentrated semen specimen is obtained for AIH.

The man is asked to collect the first half of the ejaculate in one sterile container and the second in another. The first half is then used for insemination. The main problem with this method is that it is literally easier said than done and a lot of manual dexterity is needed.

17. What are the advantages of AIH and IUI?

AIH into the cervix is usually used for couples who have severe difficulties with sexual intercourse. Another group who can benefit from this technique are men having to undergo intensive chemotherapy — they can "bank" a sample of semen in case their treatment causes infertility.

AIH is not very useful for couples in whom the man has a low sperm count since natural intercourse can achieve the same thing.

The main advantage of IUI is that is the cervix is bypassed, which is useful if there is a cervical problem (Figure 13.4). When IUI is used by itself in cases in which the man has a low sperm count, the success rates vary. Some doctors have reported good results with the procedure while others have found that the prospects of pregnancy are not increased. It may well be that it is close monitoring of the time of ovulation, rather than the IUI itself, that is responsible for any improved success rates.

One variation of IUI that does seem to be effective for patients with unexplained infertility or low sperm counts, is combined superovulation and IUI. This means that the woman is given gonadotrophins to stimulate several follicles to develop, ovulation is closely monitored and when the largest follicle has a diameter of 18-19 mm, an injection of hCG is given and IUI performed 38 hours later. The main problem with this approach is an increased chance of multiple pregnancy and most clinics would advise that if more than four large follicles develop, the cycle is abandoned or else the patient convert to some other form of assisted conception such as IVF, GIFT or POST.

18. Why do sperm have to be "prepared" for intra-uterine insemination? How is it done?

Fresh semen which is unwashed should not be used for IUI because of the risk of infection (the protective cervical mucus barrier is bypassed in IUI), allergic reactions and because chemicals called prostaglandins, which are a normal constituent of semen, cause muscular contractions of the uterus — which in addition to being painful can expel the semen sample from the uterus.

The sperm need to be specially prepared in the laboratory before use. This can be done by "washing" the semen repeatedly with special laboratory fluid and then spinning the tube containing the liquid at high speeds to remove the sperm.

"Swim-up" techniques can also be used. In these the semen is mixed with a laboratory fluid and the healthy sperm are allowed to swim up to the surface. They are then removed with a glass tube and used for insemination (or in-vitro fertilisation).

19. If a man has been sterilised, can the sterilisation be reversed?

Reversal of male sterilisation using microsurgical techniques restores fertility to a high proportion of men, depending on the way the original operation was done and provided the reversal is undertaken fairly soon after the sterilisation. If reversal is attempted many years after sterilisation, many of the men will have developed antibodies against their own sperm and so despite tubal patency being re-established the infertility is not reversed because the sperm remain immotile.

20. Can surgery help if there is blockage of the tubes which lead the sperm out of the testes?

The results of surgery depend on the site (most commonly in the epididymis) and extent of the block. In general, the results of surgery are very disappointing and only a small proportion of men go on to father children after such operations.

Sometimes the sperm can be removed with a needle directly from the epididymis. The procedure requires general anaesthesia. The sperm recovered are usually used for in-vitro fertilisation because the number is generally too small to allow successful insemination treatment.

21. What are the sexual problems that can cause infertility?

The sexual problems that may be associated with infertility are failure to have sexual intercourse, painful intercourse, premature ejaculation and impotence.

Failure to have sexual intercourse is usually the result of **vaginismus,** a term which refers to involuntary spasm of muscles which constrict the vaginal canal whenever sex is attempted. Although this can sometimes be caused by a physical problem, such as the pain caused by a tight hymen or vaginal infection, most cases result from some psychological problem. Treatment involves patient counselling by the doctor and gentle use of a series of vaginal dilators which the patient can learn to insert herself.

Painful intercourse or dyspareunia usually occurs either because of vaginal infection or endometriosis. Vaginal infection is treated with the appropriate antibiotics while the treatment of endometriosis is described in Chapter 9.

22. What causes premature ejaculation and what is the treatment?

Premature ejaculation is said to occur when the man ejaculates before the penis is inserted into the vagina.

Treatment consists of what is called the "squeeze" technique. In this method, the woman stimulates the man manually and when he feels he is about to ejaculate, she places her thumb and index and middle fingers just below the glans penis (that is, from front to back) and squeezes the penis for a few seconds. This reduces the ejaculatory desire. After a period of rest, the woman resumes genital touch, followed by the squeeze and repeats this until she can control the man's ejaculation. Once she is able to do this — usually after only a few day's practice, they have intercourse with the woman in the superior position. When the man feels he is about to ejaculate, she uses the same squeeze technique.

Over 90 percent of couples benefit from this treatment within a few weeks of starting.

23. What causes impotence and can it be treated?

Impotence refers to a man's inability to maintain an erection of sufficient firmness to impregnate his partner or complete the act of coitus.

Although a small proportion of men are impotent because of organic conditions such as diabetes mellitus, hyperprolactinaemia, previous surgery or disease of the nervous system, most cases are caused by psychological problems.

Treatment of impotence is a specialised field and requires understanding the cause, appropriate medical treatment if there is an underlying physical problem and psychological counselling by trained counsellors if there is a psychological cause. With regard to infertility, if the impotence cannot be remedied, seminal fluid can be obtained with the help of a mechanical device that stimulates the penis. Subsequently artificial insemination is performed.

15

DONOR INSEMINATION, ADOPTION AND SURROGACY

1.   What is artificial insemination with donor semen?

Artificial insemination with donor semen (AID), better known as donor insemination (DI), is a procedure to help infertile couples in whom it is not possible, or highly undesirable on genetic grounds, to use the woman's own partner's sperm to father the child.

2.   What are the indications for donor insemination?

First and foremost, DI should only be considered if both partners, after frank and open discussion, are eager to have a child by this procedure. If either partner is uncertain or opposed to the procedure then DI is not suitable for them.

The cases where DI may be considered are, first, if there is complete absence of sperm on repeated seminal analyses and treatment is not possible or has failed. Second, if the man has very diminished fertility, for example, a semen count of persistently less than 5 million/ml with poor motility, so that his chance of ever fathering a child is remote. Third, if there is a very high risk of the couple producing an abnormal baby because the man carries an abnormal gene. Fourth, if there is serious blood group incompatibility. This refers to a woman with Rhesus negative blood who has become severely Rhesus sensitised so that she would destroy the red blood cells of any Rhesus positive child within her. In such cases, if the husband has Rhesus positive blood, DI using a Rhesus negative donor may be appropriate. Finally, DI may be considered if the husband has sperm antibodies that cannot be treated.

3.   How is donor insemination performed?

The usual methods (Chapter 8, question 17) of monitoring ovulation are used to time the DI so that it is performed just before ovulation. As to the procedure itself, a speculum is inserted into the vagina to visualise the cervix and the sperm sample is then injected into the cervix. The procedure is painless.

4. Where do sperm banks get their sperm from?

Most sperm banks obtain their samples from students or other healthly volunteers (sometimes the partners of successfully treated infertility patients), all of whom have to undergo rigorous medical tests. The banks ensure that the donor's background is known and that nothing in his personal or family history would prejudice the health of the child. A minimum IQ of the donor is ensured.

5. How are the sperm frozen and how long can they be stored?

The freezing of sperm is a relatively simple procedure. A cryoprotective medium which contains nutrients and antibiotics is added to the seminal fluid. The semen samples are then drawn into fine colour-coded plastic straws which are sealed and labelled and then cooled to a temperature of minus 196°C. The straws are then stored in liquid nitrogen and are thawed when required for insemination. Semen samples can be stored in this way for years.

6. Will the procedure be confidential?

In most countries, including the United Kingdom and United States of America, DI is a confidential procedure. The name of the donor is kept strictly confidential and the recipient and the donor do not know each other's identity.

7. Will the doctor be able to select the donor to match my partner's characteristics?

Physical characteristics such as height, hair, skin and eye colour are matched as carefully as possible when choosing the donor for an individual couple. Most clinics also try to match for blood groups.

8. Is there any danger of transmitting disease through donor insemination?

There is virtually no chance of sexually transmitted infection following DI. All donors are carefully screened to ensure that there is no infection present..

9. How about AIDS?

Since AIDS became a world wide scare, it is now standard practice to advise that all semen samples be stored frozen for 6 months before they are used. The sperm donor has a blood test done before donation, and the test is repeated 6 months later. His semen sample is only used if both blood tests show that he is not an AIDS carrier. These precautions have ensured that transmission of the AIDS virus through DI is virtually impossible.

10. Can a single woman request donor insemination?
This depends on the individual clinic. Most clinics will only undertake DI for couples in a stable, happy marriage or relationship.

11. How effective is donor insemination?
DI is a very successful procedure.

Provided there is no fertility problem in the woman, the majority of women are pregnant within 6 months. The success of DI is very much related to the age of the patient. In a very large study of over 2,000 patients, it was found that the cumulative success rate after twelve cycles of treatment was 74.1 percent, 61.5 percent and 55.8 percent in women aged 26-30, 31-35 and 36-40 years respectively.

12. What is the difference between using fresh and frozen semen?
In the past, when both fresh and frozen sperm samples were used, it was found that, compared with frozen sperm, fresh semen produced a higher pregnancy rate. However, since the AIDS epidemic, it is standard practice to use only frozen sperm samples for DI.

13. Is there a risk of transmitting hereditary diseases?
Potential sperm donors are screened to ensure that they do not have a disease (or a family history of a disease) that may be passed to the woman or the baby.

14. With donor insemination are the risks of miscarriage, stillbirth and birth defects any different from those of the general population?
No.

15. Is there a risk of inbreeding in donor insemination?
This potential problem has been made negligible by restricting donors to producing only a very small number of pregnancies each, to avoid the risk of accidental marriages between DI offspring who are related.

16. Will the child look like my partner?
DI offspring are genetically related to the recipient (the mother) but not to her partner. However, as has been explained, physical characteristics are matched as closely as possible when choosing the donor for an individual couple.

17. Who should sign the birth certificate and who is considered the child's real father?
Since 1988, children born in the United Kingdom as a result of DI are, with the consent of the mother's husband, treated by law as the legitimate child of

their marriage. Before this date, under English law, a child born as a result of DI was technically illegitimate and had to be adopted by the social father.

18. We have been childless for many years. Does adopting a child "break the spell" and increase our chances of conceiving after that?
Although there are plenty of examples of couples conceiving after adopting a child, there really is no scientific evidence to support the idea that pregnancy results from adoption. It is more likely to be due to the passage of time and the accumulation of chance. Nonetheless, it is common experience that couples who desperately want to have a baby become tense, anxious and obsessive about the matter. This may affect their sexual lives, especially as they feel obliged to have sexual intercourse at certain times of the month in order to conceive, so losing all the spontaneity of love making. Once they have a child the despair and hopelessness disappear as they focus on looking after the baby. They become more relaxed, less tense and perhaps this prepares the ground for a pregnancy.

19. How does one adopt a child?
Adoption means becoming the legal parents of a child whose biological parents have decided to give up all legal rights over the child.

As a result of improved family planning methods and the availability of abortion, the numbers of children available for adoption are considerably fewer than the numbers of prospective parents. This means that, realistically, only a small minority of hopeful couples manage to adopt a child.

The first thing to do is to contact an adoption agency. There are now almost 200 in the United Kingdom. Most are part of local authority social service departments but there are also voluntary agencies (which have to be approved) that are run independently. They are often connected to particular churches. Unless you are adopting the child of a close relative, a child you have fostered for more than a year or a child from overseas, you have to go through an adoption agency. All adoptions have to be approved by the courts. Once an adoption order has been granted it cannot be reversed.

In the United Kingdom you can obtain more information from:

British Agencies for Adoption and Fostering
11 Southwark Street, London SE1 1DE

20. How are prospective couples screened?
The criteria used by adoption agencies for selecting prospective parents vary.

Most agencies prefer the couple to have been married for a few years and would not consider single parents at all. The age of the couple is also a factor and few agencies will consider the couple if the wife is over 35 or the husband over 40 years of age. The social background of the couple is important and the agency will want to ensure that the couple is able to care for the child materially as well as emotionally. Prospective parents are interviewed by social workers from the agency and have to explain why they wish to adopt a child. To ensure that the couple has come to terms with their infertility, the agencies usually ask for written confirmation from the couple's doctors that there is no prospect of successful infertility treatment for them.

The agencies try to follow the wishes of the genetic parents when they choose a family for the child. For example, some people ask that their child should be adopted by parents of a particular religion. Most agencies consider that children should be brought up in a family of the same racial and ethnic background as its genetic parents.

21. Do adopted children pose any special problems?

Contrary to the fears of many prospective adoptive parents, most adopted children grow up to be well adjusted and normal adults. There is no evidence that adopted children grow up any worse off compared with ordinary children.

22. What about surrogate parenthood?

Surrogate parenthood is a highly controversial and emotive issue that has become very topical in recent years.

Surrogacy involves a fertile woman having a baby whom she gives to the infertile couple at birth. It involves one of two procedures. In the first, the surrogate mother is artificially inseminated with the sperm of the husband of the infertile woman. In the second, the infertile woman undergoes an IVF type procedure whereby an egg is removed from her ovary, fertilised with her husband's sperm and the resulting embryo is then placed in the uterus of the surrogate mother who carries the baby through pregnancy, gives birth and then hands the baby over to the couple. This is called "womb leasing".

Surrogacy is fraught with all kinds of problems and commercial surrogacy is illegal in most countries. The problems include legal difficulties as to who bears responsibility if the surrogate mother has medical problems as a result of the pregnancy, who looks after the child if it is born with a defect and what happens if the surrogate mother forms a strong bond with the baby and refuses to hand it over to the infertile couple.

16

COPING WITH INFERTILITY

1.   Some of my friends have told me that taking a holiday will improve my chances of getting pregnant. Is this true?
At some time or other, most infertile couples wonder whether stress is causing their infertility. This is especially so if no cause for the infertility has been found or when several treatments have been tried.

The scientific evidence to support stress as a cause of infertility is, however, weak. One just has to remember that women under extreme stress, for example, those who have been sexually assaulted, may get an unwanted pregnancy and to recall that women in some third world countries who face extreme hardship, poverty and even starvation have large families, to realise that stress cannot be an important cause of infertility.

Having said this, however, if the problems caused by infertility are getting on top of you, it may well be worthwhile to have a holiday and take a break from your routine. All infertility specialists have seen couples who conceived when they were on holiday or, indeed, when they had given up trying to have a child.

2.   Can infertility treatment affect our sexual relationship?
Yes, sadly it can. It is, in fact, very common for the stress of infertility, of its investigations and treatments to throw up problems in this area.

While in the past their sexual relationship was probably a spontaneous and intimate affair, infertile couples often find that they are being asked to perform sex to order — having intercourse when the largest follicle is 18 mm in diameter on the ultrasound scan, when the basal body temperature dips, and so on. When sex becomes regimented in this way and an exercise whose only purpose is to achieve pregnancy, the ground is laid for all kinds of problems to occur. It is essential that infertile couples understand this and try not to allow it to lead to marital discord. Talking it over together is important. In some cases, it may also be wise to ask to see a counsellor.

3. Does frigidity cause infertility?

No, it does not. There is no evidence that failure to be sexually responsive causes infertility.

4. We have felt anger, guilt, frustration and depression at different times since we realised we had an infertility problem. Is this common?

Yes, we are sorry to say, it is.

In fact, it is more than a common problem; it is almost the universal experience. Infertility often leads to bouts of anger which may be directed at one's partner, the doctor, the infertility clinic or even oneself. Some people feel guilty because they feel they have brought the infertility upon themselves. Anger is often directed at people who have children, especially women who seem to have had no problem getting pregnant at all and particularly those who are going for abortions. These emotions have to be recognised as being neither unusual nor wicked; both you and your partner should realise that it is perfectly normal to feel this way sometimes.

5. Do insurance companies cover the cost of infertility and assisted conception treatment?

Unfortunately, no.

Private insurance companies do not cover the cost of assisted conception treatment.

6. Should I tell family and friends and my colleagues at work about our infertility problem?

It all depends on you and your partner. Some couples welcome and find support from those around them. Others, however, feel vulnerable, pressured and spotlighted.

7. Do you think it is worthwhile contacting an infertility counsellor?

Yes, we do.

The strains that are put on a relationship by the problems of infertility and the intrusiveness of many of the treatments can be very severe. When we add to that the reluctance many people feel to talk to relatives and friends about what they are going through, it becomes easy to see how the pain becomes magnified by isolation.

What conselling can offer in this situation is a chance to talk through your feelings and anxieties about all you are going through with someone specially trained and motivated to work in this area. In the United Kingdom, the new legislation makes it clear that infertility counsellors should not be part of the medical or nursing personnel of the infertility team treating you. It goes without saying, however, that the counsellors are well informed about the physical aspects of infertility and its treatment. Counsellors can be particularly helpful when you need to consider other options and life plans; they can also offer support to face the deep sense of loss and grief that couples experience at the prospect of continued childlessness.

8. Do all infertility clinics have counselling facilities?
We wish there were always specially trained infertility counsellors available at all infertility clinics but, unfortunately, at present this is not the case.

9. Are there any national organisations or groups to help us?
In the United Kingdom there are two national support groups that everyone with infertility problems should be aware of.

The first is the National Association for the Childless (NAC), a self-help organisation specifically for people experiencing fertility problems. NAC provides information and advice in the form of written material; there is a newsletter and the organisation holds meetings where you can meet others who are trying to cope with problems similar to your own. NAC also has a "Fertility Helpline" which you can telephone for practical advice and support. The telephone number (with a 24-hour answering service) is 021-3597539.

The address of NAC is:

National Association for the Childless
Birmingham Settlement
318 Summer Lane
Birmingham B19 3RL

phone 021-359 4887, fax 021-359 6357

The other support group is CHILD, a voluntary self-help organisation founded to help couples suffering from infertility. CHILD is devoted to improving facilities for patients with infertility, to developing counselling and to promoting research. It produces a newsletter and a series of fact sheets on various subjects related to infertility. It has a 24-hour answering service called "Linkline" (telephone number: 081-571 4367).

The address of CHILD is:

CHILD
367, Wandsworth Road
London SW8 2JJ

10.   When should we decide to "call it a day" and stop all investigations and treatment?

There can be no single answer to this question — it all depends on your particular circumstances.

On the one hand, the decision will have to take into account your age (particularly that of the female partner), the cause of infertility and the expected effectiveness of its treatment. Another crucial issue is your ability to sustain yourself during treatment. Then there is the financial burden to consider, especially if you need one of the expensive techniques of assisted conception which the National Health Service in Britain does not provide.

On the other hand, one also has to assess the availability of alternative methods of enlarging your family, such as adoption. Here, again, age is a factor that needs to be considered.

The answer, therefore, varies with every couple but we have to accept that there is a time when one should recognise that the chances of getting pregnant are so low that it makes no sense to go on. We would hope that decisions in this area would come out of discussions facilitated by an infertility counsellor.

11.   We have been told that there is nothing more that can be done to treat our infertility. What advice do you give your patients in this situation?

First, we would recommend that you get a second opinion from an infertility specialist to confirm that everything that can be done has been done. These days doctors feel much easier about second opinions than they used to and most would not forgive themselves if they had missed something curable and so denied you a chance to have it identified and put right. So we would encourage you not to be frightened of asking for a second opinion.

For many couples it transpires eventually that nothing has been missed out and that, unfortunately, nothing more can be done. In this situation adoption is a possibility and a very rewarding one too. Some questions concerning how to go about the actual procedure are answered in Chapter 15. Here we would note that in some ways adoption is the ultimate test of a couple's wish to become parents. That is because becoming adoptive parents means forgoing biological parenthood through pregnancy and concentrating entirely on the nurturing role of being a mother and a father. Adoption is therefore a solution of second choice, not a second best option.

Finally, there is the pathway of living with infertility. Not all problems in our lives can be solved and all of us, doctors and patients alike, have to remember that having children is not the sole reason for existence.

12. How does one live with childlessness?

If you have come to the end of the line of infertility investigation and treatment and feel that adoption is not for you, or not available to you, then you have reached the time when you have to try to face living with infertility.

Although it is inevitable that you will feel real grief and a sense of loss which may take time to come to terms with, this is also a time to reflect on the positive aspects of not having a child. While you may not be able to experience parenthood there are actually other joys in life. One is being able to pursue the life one chooses without the burden of looking after a child. There will be more money to spend, no necessity to find a baby-sitter every time you want to go out and you may be able to pursue a career unreservedly without having to worry how it may affect the needs of your children. You may even have the opportunity of enjoying the children of your family or friends, knowing at the end of the day, you can send them home to their parents!

As the years go by, some couples come to feel that they are fortunate not to have to experience the anxiety and distress that sometimes comes with watching children grow up and leave home. In modern society, women are able to pursue their own careers, and it is no longer "expected" that every couple will have children.

One thing, however, is certain. You are not alone. There are many couples who are sharing your experience of childlessness and who have gone on and forged rich and rewarding lives for themselves. Some may even find that the experience of infertility has brought them closer together as a couple.

Whatever the outcome of your quest to have a family, we hope you have found this book helpful. We have tried to be as comprehensive as possible but we do realise that there may be some questions that have been unanswered. If you have any suggestions or comments about this book, we would be more than grateful to receive them.

GLOSSARY

Amenorrhoea — the complete cessation of menstrual periods. A woman who has never had a spontaneous menstrual bleed in her life is said to have primary amenorrhoea. If she has been menstruating spontaneously in the past but then has no periods for 6 months or more, she is said to have secondary amenorrhoea.

Anorexia nervosa — a condition in which the person refuses to eat. It leads to weight loss and cessation of menstrual periods. ·

Anovulation   failure to ovulate.

Artificial insemination — the procedure whereby sperm is introduced into the woman's genital tract artificially instead of by natural intercourse.

Azoospermia — complete absence of sperm.

Bartholin's glands — the two Bartholin's glands are located on either side of the vagina. They secrete mucus which helps to provide lubrication during sexual intercourse.

Chromosomes — small structures within each cell that contain the genetic material that controls all the functions and characteristics of the cell. Each cell contains 46 chromosomes, except the sperm and eggs (the germ cells) which contain 23 chromosomes. The number is completed when the germ cells unite at fertilisation.

Clomiphene citrate — one of the most commonly used drugs in infertility treatment. It is used to induce ovulation. It is administered orally. If a woman does not ovulate in response to clomiphene, she is said to be clomiphene resistant.

Cumulative conception rate — a statistical method of expressing the success rate of infertility treatment which takes into account treatment success and failure as well as patients who discontinue treatment for one reason or another. It also copes with different rates of follow-up.

The cumulative conception rate gives an estimate of what the pregnancy rate would have been if all patients were followed up for the same length of time. For example, a cumulative conception rate of 60 percent at 3 months means that 60 percent of all patients would be pregnant after 3 months of treatment.

Calculation of cumulative conception rates allows us to compare the efficacy of different methods of treatment.

Cumulative live birth rate — as for cumulative conception rate, except that the end point is live birth rather than pregnancy. A cumulative live birth rate of 35 percent after 12 months means that 35 percent of patients will have had a live birth 12 months after treatment was started.

DIPI — direct intra-peritoneal insemination. It is a method of assisted conception.

Dominant follicle — the largest ovarian follicle that develops during each menstrual cycle. It is the follicle destined to ovulate.

Donor insemination — artificial insemination with donor semen.

Dysmenorrhoea — painful menstrual periods.

Dyspareunia — pain during sexual intercourse.

Egg donation — also known as ovum donation. It is a procedure in which a woman donates her eggs to another. It is typically used for an infertile patient who cannot produce her own eggs. She (the recipient) receives the eggs from another woman (the donor). The sperm used to fertilise the egg are obtained from the partner of the infertile patient (the recipient).

Electrodiathermy — an instrument which converts electricity into heat and which is used by surgeons to stop bleeding from small blood vessels. It has recently been found that by using it to burn small holes in the ovary, ovulation can be successfully induced in some women with polycystic ovary syndrome.

Embryo transfer — transfer of the fertilised egg into the uterus. Nowadays the preferred term is pre-embryo transfer.

Endometrium — the lining of the uterus. It is a specialised layer of tissue that thickens during each menstrual cycle in response to the female hormones and is shed at the time of menstruation. In the first half of the menstrual cycle (the follicular phase) the endometrium is called proliferative endometrium because it is getting progressively thicker. In the second half of the menstrual cycle after ovulation occurs (the luteal phase) the endometrium is called secretory endometrium because its glands secrete a rich mucus to nurture any future pregnancy.

Endometriosis — a condition seen in women of reproductive age in which endometrial tissue, which is the normal lining of the uterus, is found outside the uterus. It may cause infertility as well as painful menstrual periods.

Epididymis — a tightly coiled tube within the scrotum which is about 6 metres in length. All the sperm travel through it. During their passage through the epididymis, sperm acquire the ability to move forwards by themselves. The epididymis joins to the vas deferens.

Fallopian tubes — two hollow tubes which project from either side of the body of the uterus towards the ovaries. After ovulation, the egg passes down a fallopian tube where it meets the sperm. The fertilised egg then passes through the tube, enters the uterus and implants there to form a fetus.

Fibroids — fibroids are benign growths of muscle which appear in the wall of the uterus. They are very common and generally do not cause any symptoms. In a small proportion of women they may cause heavy or abnormal menstrual bleeding. Fibroids may sometimes cause miscarriage or infertility (if they are large and distort the uterine cavity).

Follicle stimulating hormone (FSH) — a hormone produced by the pituitary gland in response to LHRH released by the hypothalamus. It stimulates the follicles in the ovary to develop.

Galactorrhoea — abnormal milk secretion from the breasts.

Germ cells — these are the sperm in men and eggs in women.

GIFT — gamete intra-fallopian transfer.

Gonads — ovaries and testes.

Gonadotrophins — a collective term for follicle stimulating hormone (FSH) and luteinising hormone (LH).

Human chorionic gonadotrophin — hCG for short. It is extracted from the urine of pregnant women. It has a similar action to luteinising hormone, which is produced by the pituitary gland. It is given to trigger ovulation when the growing follicle has reached an appropriate (pre-ovulatory) size.

It is the hormone which is measured in the pregnancy test.

Human menopausal gonadotrophin — hMG for short. It is extracted from the urine of post menopausal women and contains equal amounts of FSH and LH. It is used to induce ovulation in anovulatory women who do not respond to clomiphene citrate. It is also used to stimulate the ovaries to grow several follicles in the case of in-vitro fertilisation.

Hydrosalpinx — a swelling at the end of a blocked fallopian tube.

Hyperprolactinaemia — excess prolactin production.

Hyperthyroidism — excessive thyroid hormone secretion.

Hypogonadotrophic hypogonadism — a condition in which the pituitary gland does not secrete the gonadotrophins (FSH and LH) in sufficient amounts to stimulate the gonads (ovaries and testes).

Hypopituitarism — underactive pituitary gland so that inadequate amounts of pituitary hormones are secreted.

Hymen — a thin membrane that surrounds the opening of the vagina. It is broken the first time sexual intercourse occurs.

Hypothalamus — part of the brain found in both men and women. It secretes a hormone called luteinising hormone releasing hormone (LHRH) in discrete pulses every one and a half hours in the follicular phase and every 4 hours in the luteal phase. LHRH then stimulates the pituitary gland (see pituitary gland).

Hysterectomy — surgical removal of the uterus.

Hysterosalpingogram — HSG for short. An X-ray test which involves the injection of a small amount of dye through the cervix into the uterus. It tells us about the state of the uterine cavity as well as the inside of the fallopian tubes. It is most commonly used to see if there are blocked tubes.

Hysteroscopy — a hysteroscope is a telescopic instrument which allows the inside of the uterus to be inspected under direct vision.

Immunosuppressive — something that suppresses the immune response in the body, that is, the body's capacity to reject foreign tissue.

Impotence — inability of the man to have an erection of sufficient firmness to impregnate his partner or complete the act of coitus.

Intra-uterine insemination — injection of a sperm sample directly into the uterus through the cervix.

IVF — in-vitro fertilisation, popularly known as test-tube baby treatment.

Labia majora — two large folds of skin that surround the opening of the vagina. They are part of the vulva.

Labia minora — two delicate folds of skin which lie inside the labia majora on either side of the entrance to the vagina. They form part of the vulva.

Laparoscopy — method of examining the pelvis in which a instrument called a laparoscope is inserted into the abdominal cavity and attached to a light source. It is an important investigation in infertility and is used to see if there is blockage or other problems with the fallopian tubes, endometriosis or other abnormalities in the pelvis.

Libido — sex drive.

Luteal phase — second half of the menstrual cycle after ovulation has occurred and the corpus luteum is formed. An inadequate luteal phase is one where there is ovulation but the corpus luteum does not produce an adequate amount of progesterone. A short luteal phase is one in which the interval between ovulation and menstruation is shortened to less than 10 days.

Luteal support — this refers to the administration of hormonal drugs to support the action of the corpus luteum after ovulation. The drugs normally used are hCG or progesterone.

Luteinised unruptured follicle — LUF for short. A condition in which the follicle does not ovulate but forms a corpus luteum so that the signs of ovulation such as a raised progesterone level are present.

Luteinising hormone releasing hormone — LHRH for short. It is released at regular time intervals by the hypothalamus and stimulates the pituitary gland. In some countries LHRH is called GnRH, which stands for gonadotrophin releasing hormone.

Luteinising hormone releasing hormone analogues — these are compounds in which the chemical structure of natural LHRH is slightly altered. When LHRH analogues are given they start by stimulating the pituitary gland but, with continued use, the pituitary no longer responds to stimulation so that very little FSH and LH are produced by the pituitary. The ovary then becomes quiescent. This quiescent state reverses promptly when the medication is stopped.

Luteinising hormone — LH for short, it is produced by the pituitary gland. There is a sudden increase in the amount released (LH surge) near the middle part of the menstrual cycle (approximately day 12 of a 28-day menstrual cycle) which causes final maturation of the egg. Ovulation occurs 36 hours or so after the LH surge.

Macroadenoma — also called macroprolactinoma. It refers to a pituitary tumour that secretes prolactin and which is larger than 10 mm in diameter. These tumours are always benign.

Microadenoma — also called microprolactinoma. It is similar to macroadenoma except that it is less than 10 mm in diameter.

Micromanipulation — refers to procedures devised to help the sperm penetrate the hard outer covering of the egg. It is used in assisted conception to help cases of severe male infertility.

Multicystic ovaries — a condition in which the ovaries are enlarged with cysts of 6-8 mm in diameter but with no increase in the tissue between the cysts. Multicystic ovaries normally occur in girls as they go through puberty and in women who are beginning to recover from weight loss induced amenorrhoea.

Oestradiol — one of the three oestrogen hormones produced in women. In the reproductive age group it is the most important as it has the greatest biological activity. It is produced by the ovarian follicle as it develops during the first half of the menstrual cycle and by the corpus luteum after ovulation. It causes the endometrium to become progressively thicker during the first half of the menstrual cycle before ovulation.

Oligospermia — too few sperm.

Osteoporosis — a condition in which the bones are brittle and have an increased risk of fracture. It is associated with deficiency of oestrogen.

Ovarian hyperstimulation — a complication of induction of ovulation in which there is excessive stimulation of the ovaries. There are three degrees of hyperstimulation, namely, mild, moderate and severe.

Ovaries — the ovaries contain the eggs and produce the female hormones, mainly oestrogen and progesterone. There are two ovaries, one located on each side wall of the female pelvis.

Ovum entrapment — an ill defined condition in which the signs of ovulation are present but the egg fails to escape from the ovary.

Pelvic inflammatory disease — PID for short. It refers to infection of the pelvic organs, namely the uterus, fallopian tubes and ovaries. PID may be caused by a variety of different germs and it is the most common cause of blocked fallopian tubes.

Pituitary gland — this "master" gland is located at the base of the brain and produces a large number of different hormones including follicle stimulating hormone (FSH), luteinising hormone (LH) and prolactin.

Polycystic ovaries — refers to a particular appearance of the ovaries (as seen on ultrasound scan or at laparoscopy) in which they are usually larger than normal with a smooth, thickened outer covering. The ovaries are filled with many tiny cysts and there is increased tissue between the cysts.

Polycystic ovary syndrome — is diagnosed when a patient with polycystic ovaries complains of a menstrual disturbance, obesity or symptoms of excess testosterone production, for example, acne, greasy skin and unwanted hair.

POST — peritoneal oocyte sperm transfer. It is a method of assisted conception.

Premature ejaculation — ejaculation of sperm before the penis enters the vagina.

Progesterone — this female hormone is produced by the corpus luteum after ovulation has occurred. It is responsible for the secretory changes in the endometrium which prepare the endometrium for the fertilised egg to implant.

Prolactin — one of the hormones produced by the pituitary gland. If present in excess amounts it causes milk secretion and cessation of menstrual periods in women.

PROST — pronuclear oocyte stage transfer. It is a method of assisted conception. It is the same as ZIFT.

Pulsatile LHRH therapy — a method of inducing ovulation in which small quantities of LHRH are given to the patient at regular intervals to mimic the normal pattern of release from the hypothalamus. It is used for patients who are anovulatory and who do not respond to clomiphene citrate.

Rhesus positive and negative — human blood either contains a substance called the Rhesus antigen, in which case it is called Rhesus positive blood, or it does not, in which case it is called Rhesus negative blood.

Semen — the fluid that is released at the time of male orgasm. Besides sperm, it contains fluid derived from the seminal vesicles and prostate gland.

Seminal vesicle — one of the "accessory glands" in men. It makes some of the seminal fluid. It fuses with the vas deferens to form the ejaculatory duct.

Seminiferous tubules — tiny tubes in the testes in which sperm is made. The tubules are coiled and packed together tightly. They connect up to form bigger tubes which eventually join to form a single tube called the epididymis.

Septum — a piece of tissue which forms a wall and divides a body organ, for example, the uterus, into two parts.

Speculum — instrument which is used by gynaecologists to examine the cervix and the vaginal walls.

Spermatogenesis — the process by which sperm are produced. Immature sperm cells in the testes called spermatogonia differentiate into spermatids which then turn into spermatozoa. Spermatozoa (sperm, for short) are the mature sperm.

Split ejaculate — a method of treating infertility in which the first part of the sperm ejaculated is used to inseminate the woman.

Surrogacy — a fertile woman having a baby whom she gives to another couple, usually infertile, at birth.

TET — tubal embryo transfer. It is a method of assisted conception. It is the same as TEST.

TEST — tubal embryo stage transfer. It is a method of assisted conception. It is the same as TET.

Turner's syndrome — a congenital abnormality in which a woman is born with 45 instead of 46 chromosomes. The missing chromosome is the second

X (hence the term 45 XO). It causes amenorrhoea because the woman is born with a scarcity of eggs most of which have disappeared by puberty.

Testicles — the two testicles, or testes for short, are located within the scrotum. They produced sperm as well as the male hormone, testosterone.

Testosterone — the male hormone. It is produced by specialised cells called Leydig cells within the testes.

TUFT — trans-uterine fallopian transfer. A method of assisted conception in which the fallopian tubes are cannulated through the vagina and cervix.

Unexplained infertility — a diagnosis that is made after full medical investigations fail to a find the cause of the infertility.

Uterus — the "womb".

Varicocele — a collection of dilated veins in the scrotum (like varicose veins) which, some believe, may be associated with male infertility.

Vasculitis — inflammation of blood vessels.

Vas deferens — a thick tube into which the epididymis opens. The vas deferens fuses with the seminal vesicle to form the ejaculatory duct which passes through the prostate gland and opens into the urethra.

Ventrosuspension — an operation to make a retroverted uterus (tilted backwards) into an anteverted one (tilted forwards). It is also called uterine suspension.

Vulva — female external genital organs which surrounds the entrance to the vagina. It consists of the labia majora, labia minora, clitoris and hymen.

ZIFT — zygote intra-fallopian transfer. It is a method of assisted conception. It is the same as PROST.

Zona pellucida — the tough, outer covering of the egg.

INDEX